CMOS Technology for IC Biosensor and Applications

Multi-Labs-On-Single-Chip (MLoC)

Dr. Abdullah Tashtoush

To order additional copies of this book, contact:
Xlibris Corporation
1-888-795-4274
www.Xlibris.com
Orders@Xlibris.com
136600

Table of Contents

Preface

Each year, thousands of patients in Canadian hospitals are infected with antibiotic-resistant bacteria, resulting in a cost of at least $100 million to the health-care system. Although most bacteria are harmless to healthy individuals, the symptoms of bacterial infection can be severe for patients with a weakened immune system. Outbreaks of Clostridium difficile (C. difficile) and methicillin-resistant Staphylococcus aureus (MRSA) have occurred in Canadian hospitals, leading, for example, to more than 600 deaths in Québec alone from 2003 to 2005. Early detection is critical for improved patient care and can help in minimizing the risk of cross contamination between patients. The aim of the book is to use state of the art technologies for developing handheld biosensors for pathogenic bacteria detection. There is extensive demand for a low-cost, rapid, selective and sensitive method for detecting bacteria in medical diagnosis, and food-safety inspection. Traditional methods, such as polymerase chain reaction and cell culture techniques take several hours to days to give accurate results, and require bulky, expensive equipment. In this work, we introduced new techniques for detecting bacterial pathogen cell at low concentration level based on CMOS/MEMS technology batch process. The methodology of the proposed multibiosensors that is named by multi-lab-on-a-chip (MLoC); lies on miniaturizing transducers, which is based on optical CMOS technology, charge based capacitance measurements (CBCM), electrochemical impedance spectroscopy (EIS) and CMOS microcoils incorporating with interdigitated microelectrode array (IDMA). The aforementioned approaches technically proved their capability and reliability overwhelmingly among the used conventional techniques for that reason these techniques have been proposed to create compact and portable biosensors for sensitive and rapid detection of bacterial pathogens. While the four proposed biosensors have common objectives they differ in the method and analysis used, and postulates engaged by a discipline to achieve the objectives; the inquiry of the principles of investigation in a particular field. For example, the immunosensors can smooth the progress of point-of-care testing (POCT) and become conscious state-of-the-art molecular analysis without the need of using a state-of-the-art laboratory. In addition; immunosensors reduce the cost of clinic diagnosis by miniaturizing and automate detection, and they can be categorized as capacitive, optical, electrochemical and magnetic techniques; in the light of their sensing theory.

The book includes a variety of techniques that are conducting biosensors as transducers. The single die has all of the biosensors implemented within it, which leads to a new generation of multibiosensors named as multi-labs-on-a-single chip (MLoC).

The book is organized in six chapters and four appendices. The **first** chapter includes the general introduction and discusses the problem, the objectives, the originality, the methodology, and the state of the art of the existing biosensors techniques. The **second** chapter unfolds the details behind the new design of the multibiosensors that are implemented on a single chip; this chapter focuses on the CMOS capacitance biosensor that is based on Charge-Based Capacitance Measurements (CBCM), design and simulation. The chapter then goes through the experimental setup for validating the biosensor and it ends up with some experimental results and conclusion. The **third** chapter unfolds the novel design behind the optical biosensors. These sensors were implemented using CMOSP35 technology on a single-chip that covers optical spectroscopy, VPNP design, operation, characteristics and structure. This chapter is concluded by some experiment procedures followed by the results and conclusion for the different cases for validation purposes. The **fourth** chapter expands on electrochemical impedance spectroscopy techniques for electrochemical sensing biomolecules. It details the biosensor principles, architectures and behavior, and then features the electrochemical detection techniques. The IDMA microfabrication and its characteristics, its influences and the advantages are discussed in details. Additionally, this chapter covers Non-Faradaic and Faradaic impedimetric measurements. This chapter is concluded with some equivalent circuit modeling of the immunosensor system including the experiment set-up along with some results to validate the system and a conclusion. The **fifth** chapter describes CMOS Microcoils, and magnetic field manipulation techniques. A CMOS IC microcoil array architecture and design is shown and discussed followed by a detailed description of the digital design of the control circuit and impedimetric biosensors based on CMOS technology. Moreover, the behavior and characterization of microcoil using the impedance concept and the equivalent circuit modeling of the immunosensor system is demonstrated along with some experimental setup protocols to validate the system and the chapter ends up with the conclusion. The **last** chapter summarizes the overall conclusions for the whole system. It also demonstrates the contributions and suggestions for future works and challenges a long with useful information about Labview programming and code source, and experimental procedures' images for (MLoC) system.

Chapter 1 - Introduction

Biosensors are analytical devices that combine a biologically sensitive element with a physical or chemical transducer to detect the presence of specific compounds selectively and quantitatively. This book explores the feasibility of microelectronic techniques in a successful attempt to get huge cost savings in mass production, fast reacting, and disposable biosensors [1]. Biosensors can be sorted by their input signal domain, physical and chemical biosensors. Physical biosensors include optical, magnetic, thermal and mechanical sensors. The chemical biosensors can be divided according to the transduction mode. In biosensors, natural materials are coupled to physical transducers.

Biosensors can also be categorized according to the production techniques. A microsensor is a device requiring microfabrication technology. Microfabrication is used by the semiconductor (electronics) industry to produce integrated circuits (ICs). As Bergveld showed in 1970 [1], design and packaging are important in the development of electrochemical "minisensors". They are even more crucial in manufacturing micro- and nanosensors. These biosensors are characterized by their small active sensing areas, while the size of the chip is still in the macroscopic range. Subsequently, these sensors can be Solid-state, integrated, planar, and smart sensors. The sold-state sensor refers to the device that deals with the response in the solid. The integrated sensor is made using the bulk of the silicon, while the planar uses the surface of the silicon. Therefore, the combination of the integrated and the planar produces the smart sensor often called the intelligent sensor [2]. The high Signal-to-Noise Ratio (SNR) and the electromagnetic interface characteristics made the smart sensor the best technique to implement biosensors. Semiconductors rapidly became on high demand to mass-produce these miniature devices at very low cost compared to conventional methods.

There is a strong demand for biosensors in the food production industry to follow the various steps in production, and control the quality of the final products. Therefore, the biomedical sector constitutes a potential market for biosensors, in most of life's aspects. Biosensors that are based on the enzymes that act as catalyst sensors were used to be studied and commercialized for the requirements of biomedical analysis. For instance, the glucose oxidize was the first electrode that is used to determine glucose in blood and urine for the diagnosis of diabetes. Other biosensors use either enzymes or antibodies to determine neurotransmitters, hormones and other metabolites. An implantable biosensor system is disclosed for determining levels of cardiac markers in a patient to aid in the diagnosis, determination of the severity and management of cardiovascular diseases [3]. It does provide access to precise regions of the human body, without consuming, or removing, biological fluids. Implantable biosensors yield immediate results, which are extremely useful if rapid decisions are to be made, for example, during surgery [4].

A biosensor in most general cases is constructed from a combination of a bioreceptor; the biological component, and a transducer; the detection method. The main function of a biosensor is to transform a biological event into an electrical signal. Figure 1-1 represents the principle of the operation of a biosensor, which is starting from the analyte that can provide all the information needed for its evaluation. This information can be processed and stored for later use. The process of the analysis is starting from the analyte, which is identified by the first connection of a biosensor named "the bioreceptor".

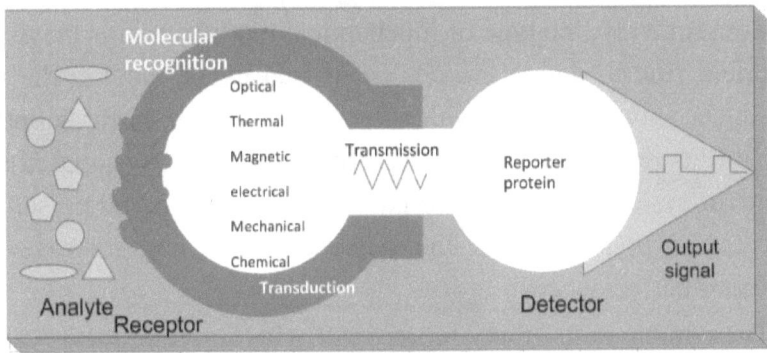

Figure 1-1 General Model for Biosensors, differentiating between molecular recognition, transduction and data processing.

The second stage of a biosensor is the transducer that takes advantage of the biochemical modification of the substrate by the bioreceptor through transforming it into an electrical signal.

Table 1.1 Common Biological Recognition Elements.

Biological Element	Mechanism for Recognition
Antibodies and antigens	Based on the specific and high-affinity antibody-antigen binding interactions to generate a detectable signal.
Biomimetric receptors	Genetically engineered biomolecules RNA and DNA aptamers.
Enzymes	Alteration of an analyte to induce or generate a signal that can be detected by the transducer.
Non-enzymatic proteins	A protein that produces a signal through a transmembrane ion channel leading to activation system.
Nucleic acids	Detection of specific DNA sequences by hybridization.
Whole cells	A substance-dependent boost or embarrassment of microorganism respiration.

Consequently, the type of biochemical modification is playing an important role to define the choice of transducer. Having the right transducer should comply with some requirements; such as optimal use of the product of the bioreceptor and give a signal that is sensitive, easily monitored, and has minimal background noise. Low background noise reduces the detection limit and improves the biosensor performance.

The combination of any bioreceptor with any transducer leads to a large number of biosensors. Table 1.1 summarizes the state of biosensor research as a function of the different possibilities of coupling between various bioreceptors and transducers. Table 1.2 demonstrates how it is possible to classify biosensors with respect to either the bioreceptor or the transducer employed.

Table 1.2   Design Parameters for Selecting a Transducer for a Biosensor.

Parameter	Definition
Sensitivity (S)	$S = \frac{\Delta y}{\Delta x}$ where Δx is the input of the biosensor and Δy is the output
Linearity	Linear system; $y = Kx$, Nonlinear system : $y = f(x)$.
Working range (W_R)	$W_R = V_{max} - V_{min}$ values that can be measured by the biosensor.
Accuracy (A)	$A = M_v - A_v$; the M_v = measured and A_v = actual values.
Repeatability	The variation in reading under the same condition.
Resolution	Minimum detectable signal.
Output	Voltage signal is preferred due to readily gather the data with no extra hardware that may increase the source of errors.
Response time	The response time is measured from the start of an input change till the output stable.
Bandwidth	The output of a physical transducer is dependent on the amplitude and frequency of an input signal.

Considering that molecular recognition generally uses well-defined reaction types and that the detection method may be extremely varied, it is logical that biosensors should be classified primarily as a function of the bioreceptor used. On the other hand, using the classification by bioreceptor is worthy and trustful because this component determines the primary action of the biosensor. Nevertheless, for the laboratory that only deals with enzymes, a classification according to the transducer employed optical, electrochemical, thermometric, magnetic, can be used [5].

The recognition process of an organic or inorganic substrate by a receptor-molecule generating a host-guest product is considered as the key to the design of a chemical or biochemical sensor as shown in Figure 1-2. The biosensing system used in this work for biological detection is a chemical sensor making use of biological components as a sensing interface. A biosensor is made of two components: a receptor and a detector. The receptor senses the variation on the surface and then converts the difference to a measured electrical signal as shown in Figure 1-3.

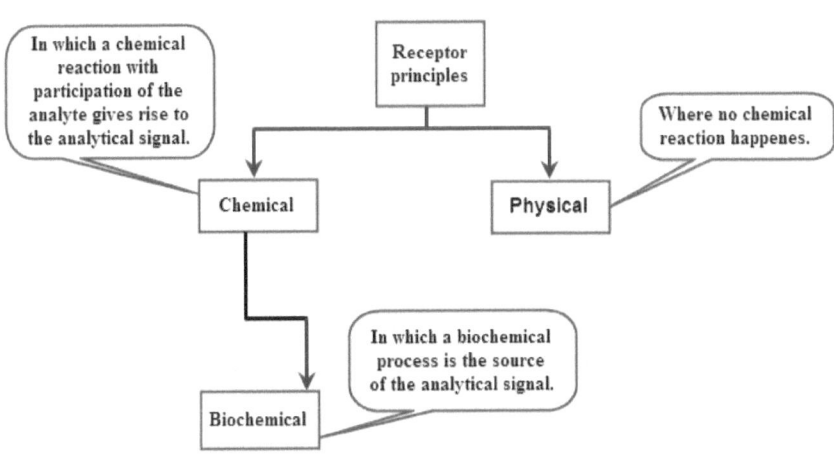

Figure 1-2   The organization chart of receptor principles.

One of the main biological recognition elements is the enzyme, which are proteins that catalyze chemical reactions where they are reacting reversibly. Biosensors are a subgroup of chemical sensors where the detection of a chemical component is based on a specific interaction of this chemical component with a biorecognition molecule, being an enzyme, antibody, aptamer, microorganism, or even a whole cell. This biological sensing element is integrated with or is in intimate contact with a physicochemical transducer [6].

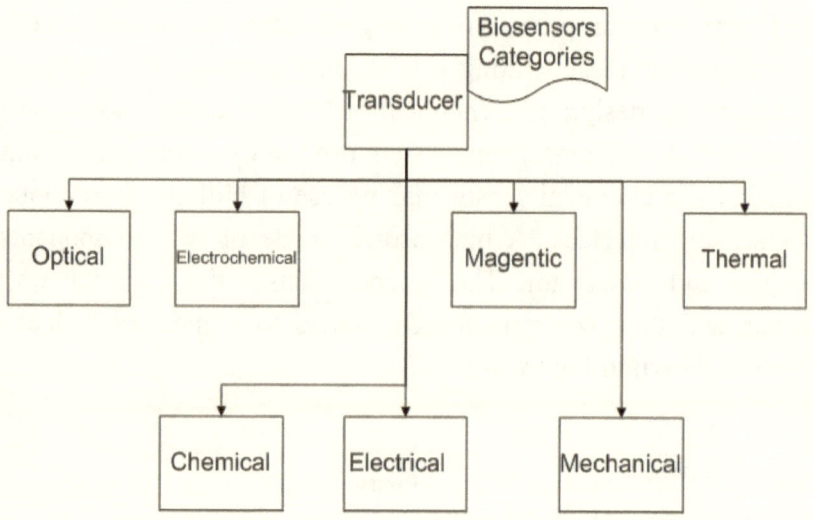

Figure 1-3   Biosensors categories.

A wide range of transducers is available to detect the interaction between the analyte and the biorecognition molecule and convert it into an electronic signal. Electrochemical, optical, thermal, and mass sensitive transduction mechanisms have been used in biosensor development over the past decade [7]. Figure 1-1 illustrates the general Model for Biosensors. A high selectivity and specificity, a relatively low production cost, a limited sample preparation time, and the potential for miniaturization are the main advantages of biosensors over conventional analytical methods [8]. Although, the healthcare industry and its high demand is pushing forward the development of biosensors, there have been many suggested applications in food, bio-processing, agriculture, and environment [9].

During the evaluation phase, often only direct cost reductions and investments are considered. Because investments are often significant, the benefits are not always completely seen at early stages of the project, therefore standoff detection techniques [10] are required. Standoff detection technologies are a sensing performed in real time that involves decision making at a distance within a certain period. Real-time standoff biological sample detection is at this time playing an important role in life science applications and medicine [11]. The principal advantages of standoff detection techniques are the reduction of the analysis time, reduction of the cost of analysis, shortening of the release time, and, as a consequence, lowering of production costs. Additionally, operators can improve their process understanding, control of the process, and, as a consequence, the first time quality because of improved product consistency.

Recently, sensor technology is applied in every aspect of life so that considerable efforts are given to improve the performance of the biosensors and reduce the cost of production. Biosensor technology also benefits from the fast growth of the microelectronic industry, which results in advanced biochips by combining the knowledge of the microfluidic with microelectronics [12]. Although the performance of a biosensor is evaluated based on a particular application, one should address the basic performance criteria in the design of successful biosensors such as sensitivity, detection and quantitative determination limits, selectivity and reliability, response time, high sample throughput, reproducibility, stability, and lifetime. In addition, the complete biosensor should be cheap, small, portable, and easy to use [13].

The biosensor must also meet requirements connected with the measurements itself; these are repeatability, reproducibility, selectivity, sensitivity, a linear region of response, and good response time [14]. Measurements have good repeatability if two sets of results obtained by the same operator, using the same sensor in the same sample are close to each other. The method is reproducible if workers in other laboratories can obtain previous results. For commercial purposes, the biosensor should have high reproducibility.

Biosensors are also categorized in terms of their ability to recognize a single compound among other substances in the same sample. This specificity quality is defined by the strength of the interaction between a molecular probe (e.g., antibody) and an antigen (target analyte) as estimated by the dissociation constant K_d. The smaller the K_d the higher the specificity of binding. Specificity is often impossible to obtain, and so the term selectivity is used [15]. Selectivity can be estimated from dose responses of a biosensor to different analyte; i.e. bacteria, which means that an interfering species responds with the same type of signal. A sensor is more selective when the number of interfering compounds is low. The selectivity of biosensors is determined by both the bioreceptor and the method of transduction. Selectivity and specificity are related to each other. High selectivity means that the contribution of an interfering species to the signal relative to the primary analyte is minimal. Specificity, on the other hand, characterizes the unique property of a bioreceptor [16]. The sensitivity of a sensor is given by the change in its response as a function of the corresponding change in the quantity being monitored. Biosensors are more convenient to use if they exhibit a linear relationship between the variation in the amplitude of the output, ΔV_o, and the input, ΔV_i as described by equation below:

$$S = \frac{\Delta V_o}{\Delta V_i} \qquad\qquad (1.1)$$

The linear region of a biosensor is obtained from a calibration curve of its response to different analyte concentrations. A good calibration curve also indicates the stability of the response of the biosensor, which should neither drift nor oscillate with time. The response time of the biosensor gives a measure of how quickly it responds to a variation in the concentration [15].

1.1 Biosensors Techniques

In biosensors where, in principle, the transducer plays a physical role and the bioreceptor has the task of molecular recognition. The information decoded by the bioreceptor is converted into an electrical signal by the transducer using measuring techniques like potentiometry, amperometry, thermometry, or photometry, all of which are based on the variation of physical quantities. The method chosen must be simple and of a reasonable size, so that it is cheap and easy to use.

The detection part in the biosensor can be achieved using various techniques, such as optical, capacitive, magnetic, and Electrochemical Impedance Spectroscopy (EIS). The selection of detection technique relies on the nature of the application and the accuracy of the analysis requested. In most general circumstances, these are the major principles techniques for analyte detection. The following section presents a brief introduction to the most widely utilized detection methods employed in biosensors.

1.1.1 Optical Techniques

Spectroscopy was originally the study of the interaction between radiation and matter as a function of wavelength (λ) [17]. Optical sensors make use of the effect of chemistry reaction on optical phenomena, such as Fluorescence spectroscopy, which is a sort of electromagnetic spectroscopy, which analyzes fluorescence from a sample. It involves using a beam of light, usually ultraviolet light, that excites the electrons in molecules of certain compounds and causes them to emit light of a lower energy. The most popular detection method is laser-induced fluorescence (LIF) for its high sensitivity [18], and absorption spectroscopy, which is a technique in which the power of a beam of light measured before and after interaction with a sample, is compared. Specific absorption techniques tend to be referred to by the wavelength of radiation measured such as ultraviolet, infrared or microwave absorption spectroscopy [19], and chemiluminescence technique, which is a technique that refers to the emission of light from a chemical reaction; that was first coined by Eilhardt Weidemann in 1888. [20].

1.1.2 *Electrochemical (EC) Techniques*

So far, optical techniques; particularly LIF detection is the most widespread detection method used in the industry. However, its major drawback is so clear in which most compounds are not naturally fluorescent, thus further steps are required to change the separation properties of the analytes. Moreover, the high cost and large size of the instrumental set up of the LIF detection are sometimes incompatible with the concept of micro total analytical systems (μ-TAS) [21], especially with the applications when portability and disposability are necessary, such as point-of-care or in-situ analysis. This is quite the opposite of the electrochemical (EC) technique [22], it is preferably suited to miniaturization, biomedical and biological samples analysis. CMOS technology that is compatible with MEMS devices allows fabrication of biosensor devices such as microelectrodes on a single chip. Consequently, it is leading to a fully integrated system. The principle transducing that is based on the electroanalytical chemistry can achieve more than one method, for instance, potentiometry, voltammetry, and conductometry [23]. Therefore, electrochemical technique is considered and it attracts a large number of scientists and researchers. The Electrochemical Impedance measurements expressed in terms of a magnitude, Z_0, and a phase shift, φ and plots in either Nyquist or Bode plot. Nyquist Plot can be obtained using the expression for $Z(\omega)$ that is composed of real and imaginary parts, by plotting the real part on the X-axis and the imaginary part on the Y-axis of a chart. The major deficiency of Nyquist plots is that it cannot enlighten what frequency was used to record a specific point. Therefore, an alternative method to analyze the data of EIS based on the Bode plot is used. Unlike the Nyquist plot, the Bode plot does show frequency information, which shows on the X-axis the plotted logarithmic values of the frequency (ω) and shows on the Y-axis both the absolute values of the impedance ($|Z| = Z_0$) and the phase-shift. Bode plots have a logarithmic axis for frequency, and magnitude is expressed in decibels (dBs). Figure 1-4 shows the general Nyquist plot [24].

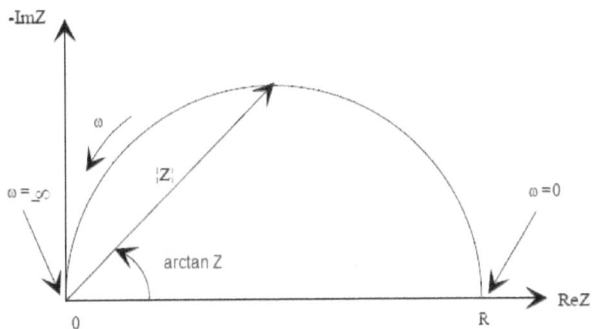

Figure 1-4   Nyquist plot illustrates the characteristics of the impedance.

1.1.3   Microfluidic channel fabrication

Biosensors is working along with microfluidic functions that can be readily integrated on microchips; using surface and bulk silicon structure with some materials that are compatible with biological issues, such as PMMA, and PDMS. High-performance detection is strongly requested. Consequently, the final success of a μ-TAS is highly determined by the ability of researchers and engineers to realize detection methods that utilize the advantages of reduced diffusion lengths and confined geometries, while also solving the challenges imposed by such miniaturization [25].

Microfluidic channel fabrication depends on master molds. Fabrication of master molds is the key to the replication technologies. There are three methods that are utilized for master molds fabrication, including micromachining methods [26], electroplating methods [27] and silicon micromachining methods [28]. After master molds have been fabricated, several methods can be applied for the replication step, such as hot embossing, injection molding and casting [29]. Creating a master requires basically couple of technologies, soft-photolithography and rapid creation of a master prototype, these are the most common methods that's employed to achieve off-chip biosensor, on-chip sensor can be done using post-CMOS process, which adds more complications to biosensors development. Soft-photolithography is a set of non-photolithographic methods for replicating patterns. A cleanroom protocols are not essentially requiring for the soft-photolithography methods for replication resolution in micro scale [30].

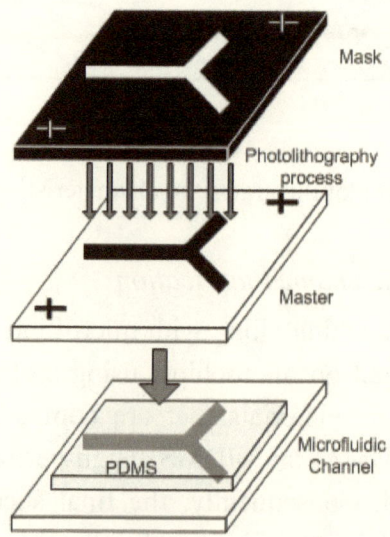

Figure 1-5   Microfluidic channel fabrication using photolithography and Rapid prototyping techniques

The second technique is rapid prototyping begins with creation of a design for a device in a using Electronic Design Automation tool (EDA) like Cadence program for example. Then; the design conveys on to a glass "Mask" using high-resolution mask aligner, which lately uses in contact photolithography to produce a pattern of photoresist. Then polymeric substrate such as PDMS is spread against the master made of patterned photoresist, to form the desired device. Figure 1-5 shows the microfluidic channel fabrication using soft-photolithography and rapid prototyping techniques. There are some requirements as mentioned in details before, but for microfluidic detection compared to those of conventional analytical systems. If we put the tremendously small volume and the cell size into account, a higher sensitivity and special structures are strongly required. As a result, the time that passes the channel would be short so the detector should have faster response times.

1.2 Biosensors instrumentation and CMOS Technology

In terms of instrumentation, a biosensor is defined as a measuring device that exhibits a characteristic of an electrical nature (charge, voltage or current) when it is subjected to a phenomenon that is not electric. The electrical signal it produces must carry all the necessary information about the process under investigation. Under this definition, a sensor could be regarded as a transducer as long it is capable to transforms one physical quantity into another. This idea is restrictive because a transducer is a quantitative device; a sensor actually possesses a much larger capacity. First, it should recognize the phenomenon, in a specific way if possible, and must translate it into a quantifiable property, which is then transformed into an electrical signal by a transducer. Thus, the original event is represented as an electrical signal and modern techniques of data collection and control can be applied [31]. In a biosensor, the phenomenon is recognized by a biological system called a bioreceptor, which is in direct contact with the sample and forms the sensitive component of the biosensor. The bioreceptor has a particularly selective site that identifies the analyte. Most biosensors make use of existing transducers and the instrumentation already associated with them. The principal modifications are made to the part of the transducer where the biological system is to be situated. Biological systems must be renewed periodically to maintain an optimal activity and the membranes that carry proteins and other reactive substances are much easier to handle if they are removable or disposable components [32]. The choice of biosensor is often related to the cost of the instrumentation for a given application. Biosensors will be used more extensively in health care in the future, if their total cost, including the instrumentation, is not excessive. In this respect, electrochemical biosensors appear to be well placed, requiring apparatus that is both simple and small. Optical biosensors generally require much larger apparatus with systems of lenses, mirrors, monochromators, and photomultipliers. All biosensors need a recording system to observe the reproducibility of the signal. This also indicates the nature of the response curve and detects any irregularities. Furthermore, it provides a permanent record of the behavior of the biosensor during both calibration and the determination itself [33].

Microsensors can be in microelectrodes, nanoelectrode, and ultramicroelectrode size [34]. The name "microsensor" means that the size of the active sensing area is in the micro range, whereas the sensing device itself is much larger and designed so that it can be handled easily. Miniaturization may result in a stronger device, such as the voltammetrically operated ultramicroelectrodes [35]. Despite the fact that the dimensions have been dramatically reduced by several orders of magnitude, the total amount of information may be greater. In the case of biomedical sensors, increasing the information gathering capability per unit volume is often the motivation for integrating electronics in the system. Integration also results in some very promising properties, besides the resulting system is more versatile, it allows drifts to be corrected; fitting and calculation software to be implemented for the measurement based on nonlinear calibration functions; and interferences to be compensated by using sensing arrays. Merging sensing elements with electronic devices for transduction and readout has led to new capabilities, but has also imposed some constraints on the biosensor system; the size of the biomolecular samples [36]. Smaller sensor and sensing layer areas is highly request to improve their performance by reducing distances between electrodes, thanks for miniaturization and Nanotechnology. For these electrodes, sensitivity refers to the decreasing surface area exposed to the target analyte. For that reason, ultramicroelectrodes are often used in spectroelectrochemistry [37]. The thickness of the sensing layer in biosensor is a figure of merit. In optical transmission sensors, however, the optical path length is equal to the thickness of the optical sensor (optode) membrane. In optical bulk membrane, technology the optical sensing layer equilibrates with the target analyte in the sample phase. Therefore, the thickness of the sensing layer determines not only the speed of equilibration, but also the optical path length. So reducing the thickness of the sensing layer also increases the sensitivity [38].

1.2.1 Immobilization

In biosensors, functionalization the surface of the bioreceptor is very important step to be occurred in order to integrate the selected biorecognition elements. This is one of the most critical steps in biosensor development because biosensor performance (sensitivity, dynamic range, reproducibility, and response time) depends on how far the original properties of the bioreceptor are kept after its immobilization. Therefore, bioreceptor requires direct or indirect immobilization on transducers to ensure maximal contact and response. Immobilization technique used for the physical or chemical fixation of cells, organelles, enzymes, or other proteins such as monoclonal antibodies, onto a solid support and solid matrix or retained by a membrane, in order to increase their stability and make possible their repeated or continued use. Immobilization has the advantage of stabilizing the protein so that it can be used repetitively. The sensing properties of a sensor depend on the physical-chemical environment of antibody and antigen-antibody complex, which are in turn determined by antibody immobilization techniques such as adsorption techniques [39], entrapment [40], cross-linkage [41], or magnetic microbeads [42].

Functionalizing the surface of the biosensor; glass or silicon by a chemical material such as epoxysilane, polylysine or aminosilane; facilitates bonding the biological recognition elements such as enzymes [43], antibodies [44] or reporter genes [45]; to the surface; i.e. polymer, glass or silicon of the biosensor.

1.3   What Multi-biosensors on a single chip all about?

By far, the main pathogen detection methods use DNA microarray techniques. These methods rely on Petri culture, colony counting and Enzyme-linked Immunosorbent assay (ELISA); which also rely on antibodies or nucleic acid polymerase chain reaction (PCR) detection [46]. The reason for this is the high selectivity and reliability of these techniques, which have different strengths and weaknesses. Culture and colony counting is the oldest method and is the one that is generally considered as the reference. It enables the detection of viable cells, but it is labor intensive and takes up to several days to obtain results. Biosensors are relatively new players in the pathogen detection arena and the use of biological recognition element generally limits their performance. Such recognition elements are mostly antibodies or DNA sequences. While DNA based methods are excellent for their selectivity and long-term stability, they usually are unable to discriminate between viable and non-viable cells. Furthermore, antibody based biosensors are generally very expensive to produce and may suffer from cross binding of other bacteria, which would lead to false results.

Miniaturization of biosensors is one of the recent trends aiming towards both increased performance and portability along with low cost for mass production. To do so, all the geometric and operational parameters have to go through proper optimization. However, it is both time-consuming and costly to study the effects of those parameters on performance by conventional prototyping. The modern approach of numerical prototyping is formulating mathematical models that best describe the system and use powerful computers to find the optimum design parameters. This does not only cut the cost of experimentation by reducing the number of experiments needed to analyze a particular problem, but it can also be used to explore problems that are difficult or expensive to test and make extrapolation to the uncultivated regions. Developing and producing miniature analytical instruments and devices can achieve a number of advantages; besides rapidly analyzing extremely small amounts of substance, it can also perform on-site analysis and analysis in security areas. Micro/Nanochip analytical devices that lead to multi/single Lab-On-A-Chip devices are microdevices that merge microfluidic technology with electrical and/or mechanical functions for analyzing tiny volumes of biological sample. Analytical microdeivces can perform a progress through two ways to produce more versatile and smaller instruments. Firstly, developing the entire miniaturized systems in which they are capable and attractive devices for the analysis of pico-, femto-, and atto-molar quantities of biological and biomedicine samples, and secondly, developing dedicated systems by accelerating the development of chemical sensors, sensor arrays, and microsensors. In addition, miniaturization might be able to produce an instrument combining or hyphenating miniaturized single elements based on different working principles without sacrificing their versatility.

The combination of both the surface-bound antibodies for identification and the surface interaction for detection process is the mechanism of the conventional detection techniques. This technique has limitations because of the inadequate biomolecular binding to the sensing surface. This is because the biomolecular binding is too small to move from the suspension and bind to the functionalized sensing surface. Recently; the specification and the behavior of the biosensors overcame this serious issue due to their high sensitivity, specificity, selectivity and improved accuracy. Therefore, the multi-lab on a single chip technology (MLoC) enhanced the modern detection techniques by including capacitive (CBCM), optical, electrochemical (EIS) and magnetic techniques all on one single chip. CMOS/MEMS technologies, integrated microfluidic channel, sorting, and biomolecular cells identification on a sort of substrates such as glass, polymer or plastic are the basis of modern biosensors (i.e. MLoC, micro total analytical systems (μ-TAS), etc…). Note that miniaturizing of the sensing systems allows faster detection of tiny volumes of biomolecular cells than that of the macroscale analysis techniques, which in sequence facilitates the new generation of biosensors that exhibit rapid biological samples detection, leading it to be fit for point-of-care diagnostics. The performance of the biosensors should be high enough to detect pathogens at low-level concentrations of biomolecular cells, which is enough to cause a disease. Such transducers could play a significant role for monitoring contamination of water supplies with pathogens. Therefore, performing successful detection at low concentration depends on reliability, sensitivity and short timing to obtain results, which become the main characteristics of biosensors. The measurement for this low level of concentration should pass through a protocol starting from the location where the sample picks up. Then the surface goes through modification followed by the treatment that binds it onto the sensing surface until finally the system reads out the results.

The aforementioned approaches so far (the CBCM, Optical and EIS methods) required sample pre-treatment steps and signal amplification strategies, which cause some complications and challenges. Therefore, this work presents a novel microsystem that integrates a fishing system with the interdigitated microelectrodes arrays (IDMA), which may lead to highly functional and versatile biosensor systems, bacteria detection with high sensitivity, and fast-response times based on CMOS microcoil. Magnetic particles are ideal to solve both challenges at once, since the magnetic fields can easily manipulate them.

1.4   Originality

The **book** includes a variety of techniques that conducts transducers as biosensors, which produces a novel outcome. The single die has all of the biosensors implemented within it using CMOSP35 TSMC technology available through the Canadian Microelectronics Corporation (CMC), which leads to a reduction of features that enhances and improves the new generation of multibiosensors, named **multi-labs-on-a-single chip (MLoC) system** by increasing its sensitivity. Implementing **MLoC** system exhibits eminent capability to achieve high performance of detecting biological samples. The achievement of this objective depends on developing and fabricating a low-cost disposable OFF-chip microfluidic channel interface (MFCI) incorporating it with the interdigitated microelectrode arrays (IDMA) using the soft photolithography technique in the cleanroom environment that will all work along with the **MLoC** system. At the end, the MLoC system goes through testing and validation using the Labview software.

Furthermore, each single biosensor out of four has a new modification in design. For the CBCM technique, a new layer sited on top of the reference capacitor isolates it. This layer consists of two metals that protect it from any external contamination in the course of running the experiment without altering the value of its capacitance. For the optical biosensor, and in the light of the fact that the sensitivity of the optical sensor depends on the exposed area to the light, the surface increases to the VPNP phototransistor 32 x 32 arrays instead of 16 x 16 arrays, also, the chip contains all the required resistors on-chip. For the electrochemical impedance technique (EIS), all of its stages implemented on-chip includes voltage controller and signal-processing unit along with their associating capacitors and resistors. For the CMOS Microcoil biosensors technique, the entire sensor implemented on-chip includes the IDMA sited on the top of the microcoils for magnetic field manipulation. The work includes two types of IDMA; on-chip using CMOS technology for CMOS Microcoil sensor and OFF-chip on MFCI surface using soft photolithograph technique inside the cleanroom. I wrote the Labview code to thoroughly control the experiment and provide us with useful information.

1.5   Why MLoC?

The main objective of this book is to develop novel multibiosensors that integrate state-of-the-art technologies that lead to a new generation of multilabs on a single chip (MLoC). The main outcome of this work is to allow detection and quantization of biological sample using miniature devices at a lower cost. Developing and fabricating the following elements will help achieve this objective:

1.   An integrated circuit reading from an interdigitated microelectrodes array (IDMA);
2.   A low-cost disposable-type microfluidic channel, which consists of an array of interdigitated microelectrodes, will act as a sensing layer for CMOS microcoils biosensors to perform impedance measurements through the magnetic field manipulations.
3.   The integration of the microelectrode chip with a simple microfluidic channel interface (MFCI) acts as working electrode for electrochemical impedance spectroscopy measurements (off-chip);
4.   Characterization, testing and validation of the entire MLoC integrated system.

5. Test environment automation for ease to extract the measured data that the Labview software will post process and analyze.

This work introduces a novel biosensor integrating state-of-the-art technologies that will allow the detection and quantify biological cells in freshwater, food, and other biological fluids.

1.6   The Methodology

As stated, the traditional biosensor methods are labour intensive and take up to several days to obtain results. Miniaturization of biosensors is one of the recent trends aiming towards both increased performance and portability along with low cost for mass production. To do so, all the geometric and operational parameters have to go through proper optimization. Accomplishing this miniaturization can be achieved through using CMOSP35 TSMC technology available through the Canadian Microelectronics Corporation (CMC) to design and fabricate the chip. Figure 1-6 shows these prototypes and will be unfolded in the following sections.

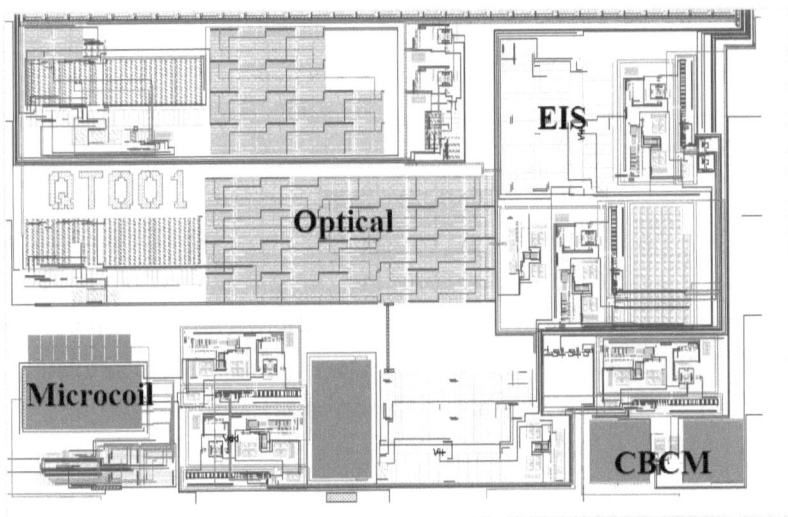

Figure 1-6   The layout of the entire biosensors devices on a single chip.

1.6.1 Research Design Strategy

Yielding the objective of this work can be reached by developing the entire miniaturized systems in which they are capable and attractive devices for the analysis of pico-, femto-, and atto-molar quantities of biological and biomedicine samples, and secondly, developing dedicated systems by accelerating the development of chemical sensors, sensor arrays, and microsensors. In addition, miniaturization might be able to produce an instrument combining or hyphenating miniaturized single elements based on different working principles without sacrificing their versatility.

1.6.2 A CMOS Resizing Methodology

Resizing CMOS transistors is a crucial step for the reprocess of analog circuits. A technology migration can be achieved by resizing the methodology that should keep or advance and enhance the original design's figure of merits, which are performance, reduction of the area of the device and power consumption [47]. The resizing methodology of CMOS transistors passes mainly through defining the features that should be maintaining, and then determining the new transistor sizes by finding the aspect ratio in the light of the results that are figured out.

1.6.3 Research tools

CMOSP35 TSMC technology available through the Canadian Microelectronics Corporation (CMC) to design and fabricate the chip was used to resize the transistors and get the technology migration from macro scale to micro scale or smaller. The experiment setup reads out the result using the Labview software. In addition, the cleanroom facilities were got involved for MEMS fabrication.

1.6.4 Data analysis

The results that carried out using Labview software from the experiment setup are analyzed and manipulated to be used for validating the system. Posteriorly; in the light of these results making decisions can be easily formed.

1.6.5   Limitations and challenges

As with any of the traditional biosensors, the MLoC system has its limitation due to the size of the biomolecular cell. Therefore, becoming familiar with the application in advance is necessary to design the biosensor but thus far, it remains a challenge for researchers in these fields.

1.7   References

[1]   Ludi, H Bataillard, P; Haemmerli, S; Widmer, Hm, "Biochemical Sensors In Industry", Sensors And Actuators B-Chemical 4 (1-2): 207-209 May 1991.

[2]   George K. Knopf, Amarjeet S. Bassi, "Smart Biosensor Technology (Optical Science and Engineering)".

[3]   Manda, Ven, Bennett, Tommy D., Yang, Zhongping, "Implantable biosensor devices for monitoring cardiac marker molecules", patent 2009.

[4]   Tran, Minh Canh, "Biosensors Sensor Physics and Technology", Series 1; publisher: Chapman & Hall, 1993.

[5]   Yuan Kun Lee, Microbial biotechnology: principles and applications, 2ed.

[6]   Liju Yang, Yanbin Li, Gisela F. Erf, "Interdigitated Array Microelectrode-Based Electrochemical Impedance Immunosensor for Detection of Escherichia coli O157:H7", Anal. Chem., 76, 1107-1113, 2004.

[7]   Graham Ramsay, "Commercial Biosensors: Applications to Clinical, Bioprocess, and Environmental Samples", Wiley-Interscience: New York. 1998. V. 304 pp, 1998.

[8]   Joseph Irudayaraj, Christoph Reh, "Nondestructive Testing of
        Food Quality", Institute of Food Technologists Series", ch11.
        Wiley-Blackwell, Number of Pages: 384, 2008.

[9]   Rajendran V and J Irudayaraj, "Detection of glucose,
        galactose, and lactose in milk with a microdialysis-coupled
        Flow Injection Amperometric sensor", Journal of Dairy
        Science, 85, 1357-1361, 2002.

[10]   Sylvie Buteau, Jean-Robert Simard, Jim Ho, John McFee,
        "Standoff detection of bioaerosols from laser-induced
        fluorescence", SPIE Newsroom, 10.1117/2.1200612.0550
        Page 2/2, the International Society for Optical Engineering,
        SPIE, 2006.

[11]   Katherine Hanton, Marcus Butavicius, Ray Johnson,
        Jadranka Sunde, "Improving Infrared Images for Standoff
        Object Detection", Journal of Computing and Information
        Technology - CIT 18, 2, 151-157, 2010.

[12]   Erickson D and D Li, "Integrated microfluidic devices",
        Analytica Chimica. Acta, 507, 11-26, 2004.

[13]   Buerk DG, "Biosensors: Theory and applications", Lancaster,
        PA: Technomic Publishing Company, Inc. 1993.

[14]   Allen, R. M. and H. P. Bennetto, "Microbial fuel cells:
        electricity production from carbohydrates", Appl. Biochem.
        Biotechnol., 1993.

[15]   Roger Breeze, Bruce Budowle, Steven E. Schutzer,
        "Microbial Forensics", pp82.

[16]   F. Baldini, A. N. Chester, J. Homola, "Optical Chemical
        Sensors", NATO Science Series II: Mathematics, Physics and
        Chemistry, Ch. 5, V.224, 2004.

[17]   Sharma, A., Schulman, S. G., "Introduction to Fluorescence
        Spectroscopy", Wiley interscience, 1999.

[18]   Laugere, F., Guijt, R. M., Bastemeijer, J., van der Steen, G.,
        Berthold, A., Baltussen, E., Sarro, P., van Dedem, G. W. K.,

Vellekoop, M. and Bossche, A., "On-chip contactless four-electrode conductivity detection for capillary electrophoresis devices", Anal. Chem. 75, 306-312, 2003.

[19]   Mohammad Ali Ansari, Reza Massudi, Marjaneh Hejazi, "Experimental and numerical study on simultaneous effects of scattering and absorption on fluorescence spectroscopy of a breast phantom", Optics & Laser Technology, Volume 41, Issue 6, September 2009, Pages 746-750.

[20]   Allen J. Bard, "Electrogenerated Chemiluminescence", ch1 & ch11

[21]   Darwin R. Reyes, Dimitri Iossifidis, Pierre-Alain Auroux, Andreas Manz "Micro Total Analysis Systems. 1. Introduction, Theory, and Technology, Anal. Chem., 74, p.p. 2623-2636, 2002.

[22]   Thevenot, D.R., Toth, K., Durst, Wilson, G.S, "Electrochemical biosensors: recommended definitions and classification", Biosens. Bioelectron 16, 121/131, 2001.

[23]   A.J. Bard, M. Stratmann, P.R. Unwin, "Instrumentation and Electroanalytical Chemistry", vol. 3, Wiley-VCH, New Jersey, (Chapters 1-2), in: Encyclopedia of Electrochemistry, 2003.

[24]   Lorenz, W.; Schulze, K. D. "Application of transform-impedance spectrometry", Journal of Electroanalytical Chemistry, 65(1), 141-153, 1975.

[25]   Katri Huikko, Risto Kostiainen, Tapio Kotiaho, "Introduction to micro-analytical systems: bioanalytical and pharmaceutical applications", Review Article, European Journal of Pharmaceutical Sciences, Volume 20, Issue 2, Pages 149-171, October 2003.

[26]   Martynova, L., Locascio, L. E., Gaitan, M., Kramer, G. W., Christensen, R. G. and Mac-Crehan, W. A., "Fabrication of plastic microfluid channels by imprinting methods", Anal. Chem. 69, 4783-4789, 1997.

[27]   Ehrfeld, W. and Munchmeyer, D., "Three-dimensional microfabrication using synchrotron radiation". Nucl. Instrum. Methods Phys. Res. A 303, 523-532, 1991.

[28]   Marc J. Madou, "Fundamentals of Microfabrication: The Science of Miniaturization, 2nd ed, ISBN-13: 978-0849308260, March 13, 2002.

[29]   Mitchelson, "New High Throughput Technologies for DNA Sequencing and Genomics, Volume 2 (Perspectives in Bioanalysis) (Perspectives in Bioanalysis)", Elsevier B.V, 2007.

[30]   Zhiwei Zou, Junhai Kai, Michael J. Rust, Jungyoup Han, Chong H. Ahn, "Functionalized nano interdigitated electrodes arrays on polymer with integrated microfluidic for direct bio-affinity sensing using impedimetric measurement", Sensors and Actuators A: Physical, Volume 136, Issue 2, Pages 518-526, 16 May 2007.

[31]   Vladimir Ogourtsov, "Electronic Instrumentation Systems", http://www.tyndall.ie/PDFs/esi.pdf.

[32]   Martin L.Yarmush, Mehmet Toner, Robert Plonsey, Joseph D.Bronzino, "Biotechnology for Biomedical Engineers (Principles and Applications in Engineering", ISBN 0-203-00903-7, Master e-book ISBN, © CRC Press LLC, 2003.

[33]   R.F Taylor, Jerome S. Schultz, "Handbook of Chemical and Biological Sensors", pages 604, ch.7, 1996.

[34]   Soledad Bollo, Claudia Yáñez, Juan Sturm, Luis Núñez-Vergara, and Juan A. Squella, "Cyclic Voltammetric and Scanning Electrochemical Microscopic Study of Thiolated β-Cyclodextrin Adsorbed on a Gold Electrode", Langmuir, 2003, 19 (8), pp 3365-3370, March 6, 2003.

[35]   Daniel Berdat, "Interdigitated Electrode DNA Biosensor for Detection of Food-borne Pathogens by Impedance Spectroscopy", École Polytechnique Fédérale De Lausanne, Book 2009.

[36]   David O. Wipf, R. Mark Wightman, "Submicrosecond measurements with cyclic voltammetry", Anal. Chem., 1988, 60 (22), pp 2460-2464, 1988.

[37]   Eyal. Sabatani, Israel. Rubinstein, "Organized self-assembling monolayers on electrodes. 2. Monolayer-based ultramicroelectrodes for the study of very rapid electrode kinetics", J. Phys. Chem., 1987, 91 (27), pp 6663-6669, December 1987.

[38]   Michael L. Simpson, Gary S. Sayler, Bruce M. Applegate, Steven Ripp, David E. Nivens, Michael J. Paulus, Gerald E. Jellison Jr, "Bioluminescent-bioreporter integrated circuits form novel whole-cell biosensors", Trends in Biotechnology, Volume 16, Issue 8, Pages 332-338, 1 December 1998.

[39]   Parida SK, Dash S, Patel S and Mishra BK, "Adsorption of organic molecules on silica surface", advances in Colloid and Interface Science, 121:77-110, 2006.

[40]   Cosnier S, "Biosensors based on electropolymerized films: New trends", Analytical and Bioanalytical Chemistry 377:507-520, 2003.

[41]   Hermanson GT, "Bioconjugate Techniques. Academic Press, London", 1996.

[42]   J. C. Rife, M. M. Miller, P. E. Sheehan, C. R. Tamanaha, M. Tondra, L. J. Whitman, "Design and performance of GMR sensors for the detection of magnetic microbeads in biosensors", Sensors and Actuators A: Physical, Volume 107, Issue 3, Pages 209-218, 1 November 2003.

[43]   Smith AL *et al.*, "Oxford dictionary of biochemistry and molecular biology", Oxford [Oxfordshire]: Oxford University Press, 1997.

[44]   John Bradley, "Immunoglobulins", Journal of Medical Genetics, 11, 80, 1974.

[45]   Becher OJ, Holland EC, "Genetically engineered models have advantages over xenografts for preclinical studies". Cancer Res. 66 (7): 3355-8, April 2006.

[46]   Ursula E. Spichiger-Keller, "Chemical Sensors and Biosensors for Medical and Biological Applications", Wiley VCH, 1998.

[47]   Levi, T.; Tomas, J.; Lewis, N.; Fouillat, P., "A CMOS Resizing Methodology for Analog Circuits ", Design & Test of Computers, IEEE, Volume: 26, Issue: 1, Page(s): 78-87, 2009.

Chapter 2 - CMOS capacitance sensor based on Charge-Based Capacitance Measurements

2.1 Introduction

The use of the industrial complementary metal oxide semiconductor (CMOS) technology for fabricating biosensors, phototransistors, Potentiostat, with the aim of reducing costs, size and time to market them will be discussed along with the implementation of CMOS-based capacitive sensors for biomolecular detection purposes. The system is implemented using CMOSP35 technology that uses the TSMC fabrication process. Note that the system consists of interdigitated capacitor structures, metal-metal comb-capacitors (MMCC), signal detection and processing circuitry. The proposed CMOS capacitive based sensors offer a number of advantages including small size, fast response time and low-cost for mass production. CMOS capacitance based systems, employed in immunosensors, plays a major role for cancer markers. This system is specifically designed, fabricated and experimentally validated.

In this chapter, the design and implementation of capacitive sensors for biomolecular detection purposes is largely discussed. The proposed system makes use of bacteriophage or phage organisms as recognition elements to detect deadly bacteria such as E-Coli and Salmonella. The system works based on monitoring the changes in capacitance signals caused when the target bacteria are attached to the sensing interface. The system consists of interdigitated capacitor structures, signal detection and processing circuitry. The signal is detected by a Charge Based Capacitance Measurement (CBCM) technique. The adopted technique was originally proposed as an accurate method to characterize interconnects capacitance in deep submicron CMOS integrated circuits [1]. The phage organisms are immobilized on the surface of the capacitor and together they form the sensing interface. The CMOS capacitive based sensors have the huge advantage of small size, fast response time, and low-cost for mass production.

Presently, much of the bacterial analyses run in clinical laboratories, which is time consuming and requires extensive professional expertise. In addition, the majority of the available commercial devices are massive, which make them not suitable for field applications. Furthermore, these commercial devices are generally growth-based, which means that the presence of bacteria has to reach a high threshold level in order to get a reading from the apparatus. The growth-based technique is time consuming as it takes from hours to days to get the results.

The technique is a real-time bacterial sensor microsystem that holds great promise for versatile applicability such as food safety, national security, and clinical diagnostics. This sensor system design falls back on the use of specific bacteriophages, which are viruses that recognize specific receptors on the bacterium surface with extreme selectivity and sensitivity. The phages bind to the surface of the bacterium and inject genetic material. Capacitive sensors offer many advantages besides their capability in their straightforward method of sensing electrode motion; they can also detect conductive, or the dielectric properties of a biomaterial site onto the sensing capacitor. For that reason, the capacitance approach measurements technology is known as a powerful technique in biosensor applications due to its tremendous capability, stability and low-noise signal in sensing process [2].

2.2 Sensor System Design

To reduce the cost and time required for the accurate clinical analysis and life science application, the biosensor based capacitance immunosensors were developed. This immunosensor for on-site screening and monitoring of contaminants determines the level of contamination by measuring the change of capacitance caused by the insertion of a biological sample to the system. The capacitive biosensor works when contaminant biomolecules bound to specific antibodies on the sensing electrode. When a biomolecular sample inserted into the microfluidic channel is embedded with IDMA as a sensing electrode, the sensing field passes through the biomaterial. The presence of the biomolecular material alters the dielectric, which alters the capacitance accordingly. The capacitance will change in relationship to the thickness or density of the biomaterial [3]. The compound dielectric constant of the bulk analyte mixture determines the capacitance. For that reason, the capacitance change can be either positive or negative depending on whether the analyte has a higher or lower dielectric constant K leading to show significant variation with biomaterial properties or with frequency. Afterwards, the measurements are recorded as a difference between sensing and reference capacitors.

2.2.1 Interdigitated microelectrodes array (IDMA)

Interdigitated array of microelectrodes is a widespread technique. For example, it is used to develop biosensors for monitoring the catalyzed reaction of enzymes, the biomolecular recognition events of specific proteins. Interdigitated array microelectrodes (IDMA) are integrated with the CBCM technique in order to miniaturize the conventional electrodes, enhance the sensitivity and use the flexibility of electrode fabrication to suit the conventional electrochemical cell format or microfluidic devices for a variety of applications in chemistry and life sciences. This work focuses on IDMA that is based on the CBCM technique as biosensors.

Interdigitated microelectrode arrays (IDMAs) are fabricated on glass wafers and optimized to obtain optimal oxidation and reduction reactions. Therefore, IDMA are utilized to increase the sensor capacitance performance in a tiny biomolecular volume.

A custom CMOS capacitance sensor is designed using the topology shown in Figure 2-1. A CBCM based capacitive sensor circuit has been reported [4]. In general, the behavior of the CBCM technique can be characterized based on the current of each branch of the CBCM circuit that is amplified by a current mirror. This current is then converted to a DC voltage using a simple capacitor (C_{int}).

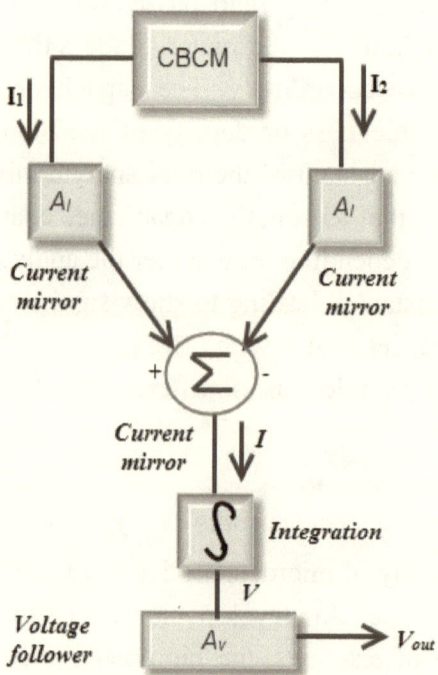

Figure 2-1   Simplified block diagram of CBCM technique.

A differential amplifier (DAMP) finally subtracts the resulting voltage outputs of both the sensor circuits' reference and sensing electrodes as shown in Figure 2-2. It is noted that the only important limiting factor on the accuracy of this sensor circuit is the input voltage offset of the DAMP circuit. The proposed biosensor boasts a fully differential architecture using sensing and reference capacitors to achieve improved resolution and high signal-to-noise ratio (SNR). The sensing and reference capacitors are identical interdigitated structures with a metal layer placed over the structure for immobilizing the phage organisms and protecting the structure against hydration.

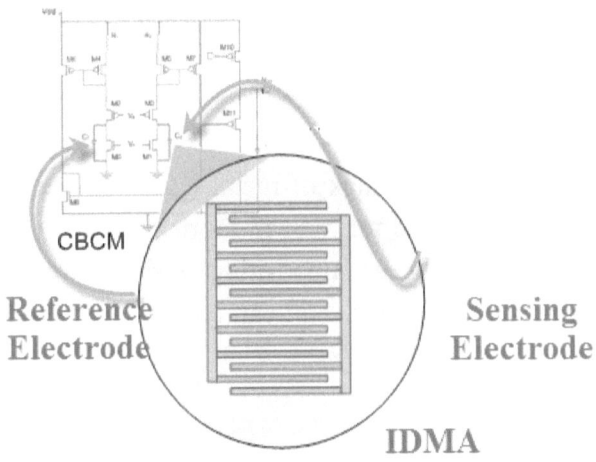

Figure 2-2   Schematic diagram of CBCM technique.

The sensor system is designed using the CMOSP35 process available through the Canadian Microelectronics Corporation. The interdigitated capacitors are implemented using the metal layer available in the CMOS process. Another metal layer is placed over the capacitor structure. A Passivation (dielectric) layer protects the CMOS circuit and the reference capacitor where only the sensing capacitor is exposed to the sample by opening the dielectric layer over it. In addition, the unexposed region of the CMOS system was covered with epoxy after the chip was fabricated as protection for use in aqueous samples. The CMOS capacitive biosensors that incorporate IDMA configurations are introduced to be used in biological and life science application in order to abuse the advantages of IDMA, which have a narrow gap between the electrodes, since the distance between electrodes is directly related to the sensitivity of the sensor. The electric field generated in one of the IDMA is distributed in the area where the target interacts with the bioreceptor, creating a change of the generated electrical field, which is detected on the second IDMA. The ionic media is a drawback in this kind of sensors because of the pre-dominant electrical spreading resistance of the solution. Figure 2-3 shows the schematic diagram of the interdigitated capacitor; named Metal-Metal Comb-Capacitors (MMCC). The capacitors are fabricated exclusively with layers and processing steps are available in the standard CMOS process. Note that the electrode E1 (Blue) is formed by metal layer one while the electrode E2 (orange) is a stack of metal layers one and two. While many of the processes used for MEMS fabrication are not compatible with the CMOS IC process, depositing a sensor material onto a previously fabricated CMOS circuit can create a very useful category of sensors.

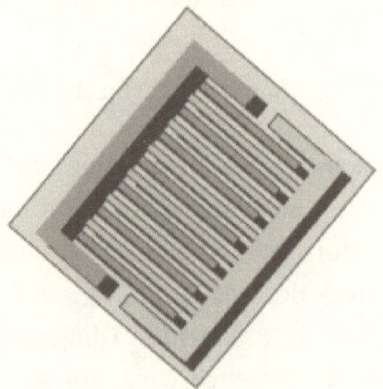

Figure 2-3   A schematic diagram of the interdigitated capacitor.

In this work, a CMOS capacitance biosensor composed of immunosensors bioreporters is reported; genetically engineered bacterial pathogen cells, are deposited onto interdigitated microelectrodes (IDMA) that are fabricated through the CMOS technology process provided by CMC. The bioreporter used for this work is immobilized on the surface of the sensor capacitance made of IDMA. The immunosensor is detected by measuring the variation of the capacitance as a function of the concentration of bacteria [5]. The interdigitated microelectrode configuration is enhancing the sensitivity of the biosensor by maximizing the sensing area with a strong electrical field due to small gap between the fingers of the capacitor [6]. Figure 2-4 shows a layout of the interdigitated microelectrodes arrays capacitor. It consists of 30 electrode pairs and occupies an area of 100.3 μm x 102.8 μm, where the interdigitated microelectrodes arrays' sensor area is similar to that of the reference electrode. However, it is noted that there is an isolation layer laid out on the reference electrode to protect it from any external contamination. The width and spacing of single electrodes are 1.0 μm and 0.6 μm respectively, as shown in Figure 2-5. CMOSP35 technology defines the height of the microelectrode and the extracted capacitance value is around 500.005fF. A capacitive biosensor utilizing a couple of capacitors are each composed of interdigitated microelectrodes array.

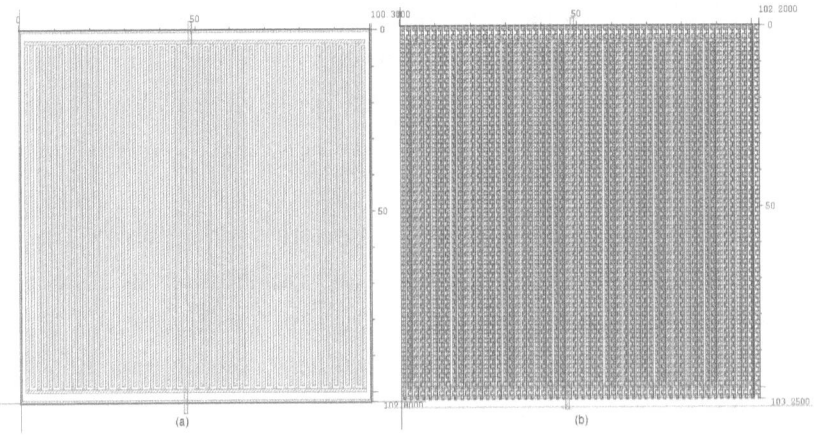

Figure 2-4   Layout of the interdigitated microelectrodes arrays capacitor, (a) the sensor capacitor (b) the reference capacitor.

The reference capacitor is covered and protected entirely where the sensing capacitor is modified and functionalized separately and chemically by a sensitive polymer. The presence of the polymer on top of the sensing capacitor aims to absorb the biorecognition elements to bind the bacterial pathogen cell. Therefore, any variation on the surface will directly change the capacitance of the electrode and thus it is electrically detected and recorded. Figure 2-6 is demonstrating the block diagram of the CBCM integrated with the Interdigitated Microelectrode array and signal-processing system, where Figure 2-7 shows the layout of the entire CMOS capacitance biosensor.

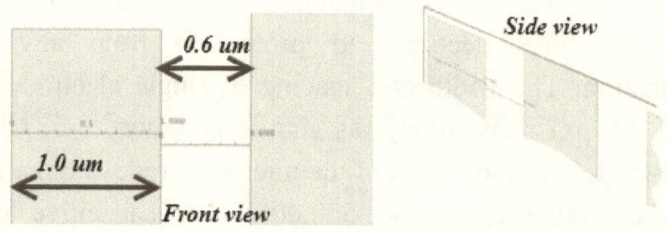

Figure 2-5   The dimension of the width and gap for the IDMA.

The IDMA technique based on CMOS technology to implement the capacitive biosensor shows an unprecedented robustness and more sensitivity owing to a large area of the sensing surface and a small electrode gap (0.6 μm) besides other known advantages of IDMA were reported [7].

Such technology allows further detection of tiny biomolecular samples in medicine and life science applications such as a label-free capacitive DNA sensing. The mechanism of this technology lies on characterizing the immunoreactions that occur on the sensing surface by capacitive parameters. As soon as the DNA targets bind on the sensing surface, the capacitance of the electrode will change accordingly. The read-out circuitry including the Labview software is monitored and recorded by the output of the sensor. The CMOS capacitance approach offers many advantages over the other techniques. Besides the high sensitivity thanks to the presence of IDMA, it is also useful in real-time detection and it costs less with respect to the optical technique expenses [8].

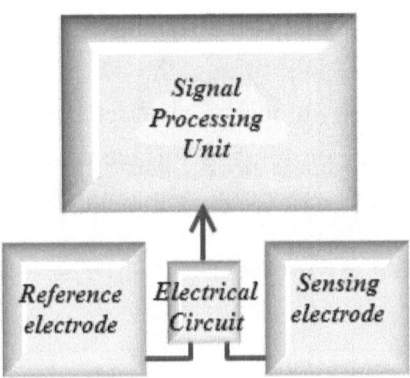

Figure 2-6   The Block diagram of the CBCM integrated with Interdigitated Microelectrode array and signal-processing system.

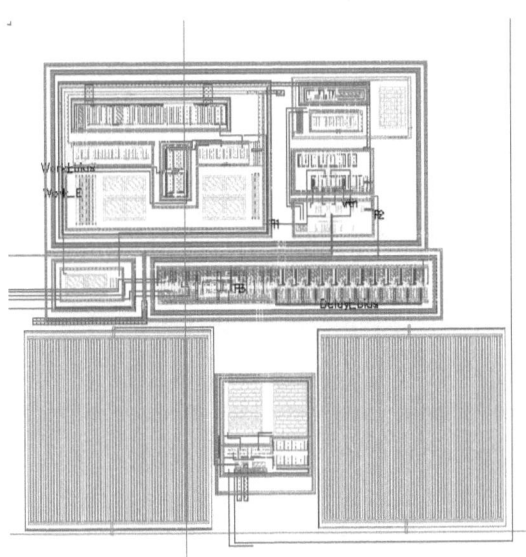

Figure 2-7   The Layout of the entire CMOS capacitance biosensor.

2.2.2 Biosensor system design and architecture

Capacitive immunosensors are based on altering electrical conductivity at a constant voltage, which is caused by immunoreactions that specifically generates or consumes ions. Fernandez-Sanchez *et al.* [9] developed a disposable, non-competitive capacitive immunosensor for PSA. This work presents femto-molar detection bacterial pathogens sensor based on CMOS capacitance technology. Figure 2-8 illustrates the entire capacitive biosensors detecting system. The binding of bacterial pathogen cells and immobilized antibodies on sensing surface produces negative charges, which form an electrode-electrolyte capacitance interface [10].

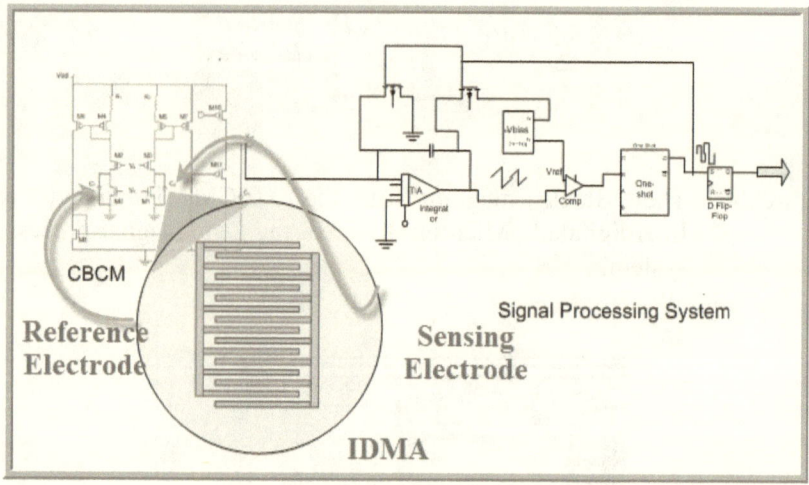

Figure 2-8   The Biosensor circuit based on CBCM.

The measurement of the changes in capacitance of the biosensor has a short response time thus allowing the rapid detection in the presence of the specific bacteria. The label-free bacterial pathogens biosensing approach is incorporated with interdigitated microelectrode arrays under an externally applied electrical field. It is no longer limited to observing the existence of the live pathogens due to the variations in characteristics of the architecture electrochemical of the actuators. It also has the capability to detect pathogens whether they are live or dead cells. Figure 2-8 shows the CMOS biosensor based on the CBCM detection approach. Note that the capacitance pathogen biosensor is based on the sensing surface with the immunoglobulin (i.e. antibodies), which provides specificity for the target bacterial pathogen. The live bacterial pathogen bound to the immunoglobulin on the electrode disturbs the surface-restricted electrical field making the capacitance between the electrodes decreases due to change the permittivity of the media. This decrease in capacitance value can be detected as the positive signal. By contrast, dead bacterial cells are not voluminous enough to induce noticeable changes in the electrical field lines distribution [11]. The microfluidic channel (MFC) that is built of interdigitated microelectrodes arrays is used as the transducer-sensing surface. Interdigitated microelectrodes arrays are capable to sense narrow changes in the electric parameters of the electrodes surface [12]. In addition, IDMA can be employed for detecting the presence of particular dielectric objects on the surface of electrodes [13]. As aforementioned, the sensing surface is interdigitated microelectrode arrays made by CMOS technology CMOSP35 providing by CMC. Thus both the resistivity "ρ" and the permittivity ε of the solution will be measured and recorded accordingly as long as they are dunk in the fluid system [14][15]. Electrolyte medium like the metallic conductor can act upon Ohm's law:

$$R_{sol} = \frac{E}{I} \qquad (2.1)$$

Where parameter R_{sol} is the resistance of the body of the solution in ohms (Ω), parameters E and I are the potential difference (V) and the current (A) respectively. By definition, the conductance G, is the inverse of the resistance R of a consistent body of uniform cross section. In the electrolyte solution, the conductance G is given by:

$$G = \frac{1}{R} = \frac{A}{l}k \qquad (2.2)$$

Where "*k*" is the *specific conductance* with units $\Omega^{-1}.m^{-1}$, *A* and *l* *are geometrical parameters*. Note that it is difficult to define accurately geometrical parameters *A* and *l*, therefore there is a need to use parameters from a known specific source and map it to the fluidic cell parameters. Therefore, the cell constant $\mathcal{K}_{cell}$ can find out as follows:

$$\mathcal{K}_{cell} = \frac{l}{A} = kR \tag{2.3}$$

Resistance $\quad R = \frac{\rho l}{A} = \frac{l}{\sigma A} = \frac{\mathcal{K}_{cell}}{\sigma} = \rho \mathcal{K}_{cell} \tag{2.4}$

Conductance $\quad G = \frac{1}{R} = \frac{\sigma A}{l} = \frac{A}{\rho l} = \frac{\sigma}{\mathcal{K}_{cell}} = \frac{1}{\rho \mathcal{K}_{cell}} \tag{2.5}$

Where; $\mathcal{K}_{cell}$ is the cell constant (m^{-1}) and can be found out by measuring the resistance R_{sol} of a cell filled with an electrolyte of a known specific conductance *k*. having cell constant $\mathcal{K}_{cell}$ then the specific conductance *k* of any solution can be determined based on practical tentative resistances values using any of the equations mentioned above. By definition, specific conductivity is the inverse of the specific resistance of an electrolyte measured between two electrodes 1.0 cm^2 in area and 1.0 cm spaced out. The higher the concentration of ionic ingredient, the higher the conductivity will be present in the system. Note that conductivity, "σ", is the inverse of resistivity "ρ"and the temperature depends heavily on the parameter.

The double layer capacitance in the electrolyte behaves like two parallel plates' theory, thus the capacitance in the electrolyte electrode interface can be given as follows:

$$C = \frac{\epsilon A}{d} = \frac{\epsilon}{\mathcal{K}_{cell}} = \frac{\epsilon_0 \epsilon_r}{\mathcal{K}_{cell}} \tag{2.6}$$

Where ϵ_0 is the electric constant equal to $\epsilon_0 \approx 8.854$ pF m^{-1} and the permittivity ϵ_r is the dielectric constant of the material between the plates. In the light of the aforementioned regarding the cell constant "$\mathcal{K}_{cell}$", the relation between the measured values of the resistance; R_{sol} and the capacitance; C can be undoubtedly noted by the direct proportion to the resistance R_{sol} and inverse proportion to the capacitance; C, (Source: PAC, 1974, 37, 499 (Electrochemical nomenclature) on page 511) the constant cell is given by:

$$\mathcal{K}_{cell} = \frac{l}{A} = kR = \frac{\epsilon}{C} = \frac{R}{\rho} \qquad (2.7)$$

For capacitive detection of bacterial pathogens, a suitable frequency should be selected under the application of a specific electrical field is needed. In the presence of bacterial pathogen binding to the surface of the electrodes via the biomolecular recognition of antibodies, the entire system will be perturbed and the variation will be detectable and measurable. In addition, the geometries of the electrodes and interface gap between the electrolyte and electrode are playing a significant role in the cell constant.

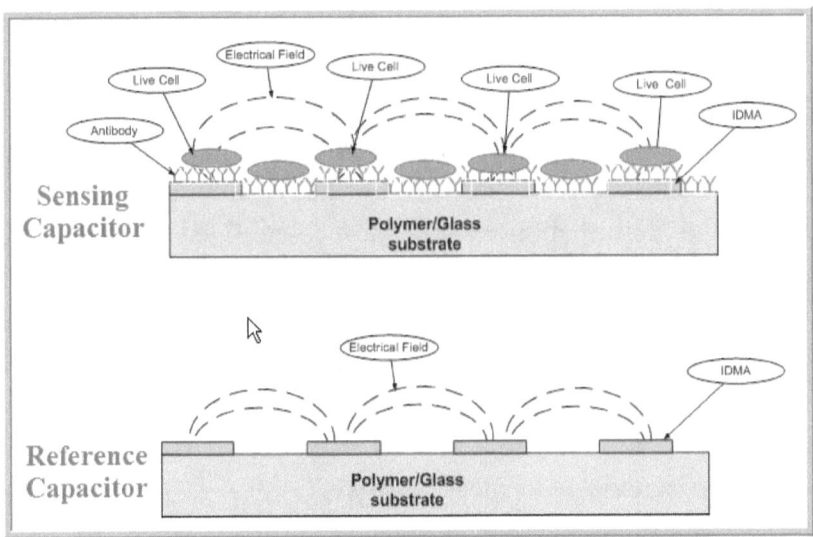

Figure 2-9   Surface sensing binding with pathogens.

As soon as the surface of the sensing transducer is modified by filling it with a biomolecular sample as a new dielectric in between the interdigitated electrodes it leads to variation in the capacitance C_T:

$$C_T = \frac{A\, \epsilon_r \varepsilon_0}{d} \tag{2.8}$$

Biosensors based on capacitance measurements incorporated with IDMA generates strong electrical field between the fingers when pathogens are detected. The mechanism of this technique depends on the generated electrical field, where it starts from one side and ends on the other finger of IDMA as shown in Figure 2-9. The electrical field is spreading in the gaps creating a disturbance in a form of a generated electric field. The latest criterion has tiny volume due to the membrane potential of cells breaks down and the ions in the cell are driven out. Dead cells still have the capability to be binding to the antibodies similar to live cells. However, their impact on variation in capacitance properties of the interface is negligible. Therefore, the plot of capacitance of the two categories will clearly distinguish between the behaviors of each criterion under the same conditions. Differentiating between the living or dead pathogen is a big advantage for the IDMA configuration. By contrast, the capacitance approach is not susceptible to these issues since the transducer can differentiate the volume of the insulating cell via the perturbation of the surface-confined electrical field measured at a proper frequency range. The interdigitated transducers have a finger width of 1 μm and the gap between fingers is 0.6 μm, and these geometries confines 80% of electric field lines and currents within a distance equal to half of the pitch [16]. Therefore, this layout makes the detection of micrometer-sized dielectric objects such as live bacterial cells most sensitive.

The target bacteria gets attached to the immobilized phages on the sensing capacitor, which changes the capacitance of the comb capacitor by interrupting the electrical field between interdigitated fingers as shown in Figure 2-9. The phages are not immobilized on the reference capacitor and hence it does not experience any capacitance changes with the changes in bacterial concentrations. The CMOS Charge Based Capacitance Measurement (CBCM) circuit measures the difference of the capacitance between the sensing and reference capacitors and provides a voltage output [17]. CMOS capacitive biosensors are used recently on different applications such as Multi-Labs-on- a chip and micro technology system. Figure 2-10 illustrates the entire system of MLoC applications.

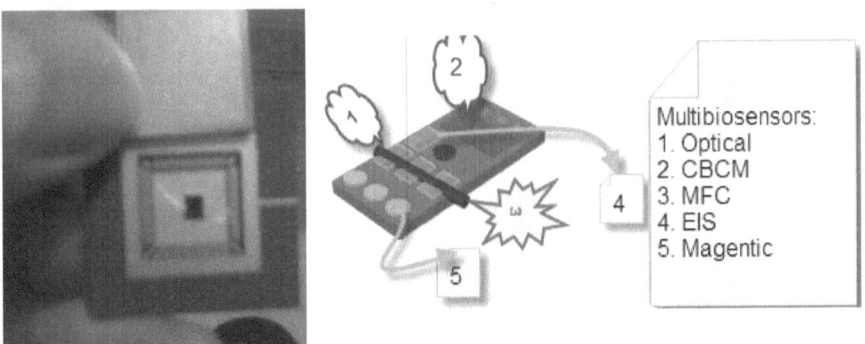

Figure 2-10 An illustration of CMOS capacitive biosensor for MLoC applications.

2.2.3 Read-out circuitry

The CMOS signal-processing system, shown in Figure 2-11 is a key component of the impedance measurements system. The CMOS circuit is designed and fabricated using the TSMC CMOSP35 processing technology. All transistors operate at the standard 3.3 V. The simplest noise approximation for the microluminometer assumes the detection of a dc signal in wide-band white noise [18].

The signal-processing circuit aims to convert the current passing through the output stage into a digital signal, where the frequency is proportional to the concentration of the pathogens in medium. This is solved by using a hybrid analog/digital integration scheme as shown in Figure 2-11. In this circuit, an analog integrator and a discriminator convert the current generated as byproduct into a train of digital pulses; current-to-frequency converter (CFC).

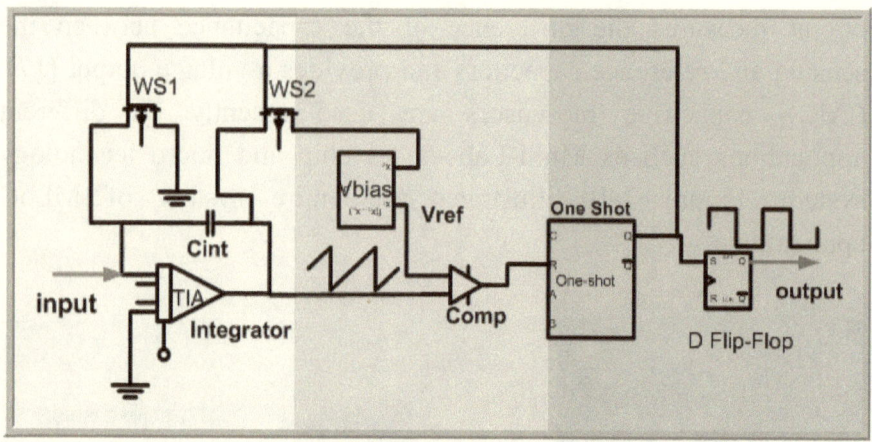

Figure 2-11 Block diagram of the signal-processing circuit.

These pulses are counted for a fixed time (t_0), and the result is a digital word that is proportional to the working electrode current intensity. This system has several advantages compared to other processing options such as fast recovery from overload, and ease of analog-to-digital conversion reported in optical detection systems [19].

The mechanism of the signal-processing system can be explained by electronically analyzing the behavior of the circuit. The key for the signal-processing circuit are switches WS1 and WS2. Initially, both of the switches are closed during the beginning of the integration process. Consequently, a bias is applied on the detector and the output of the integrator is at "ground" and 0.5 V respectively. The role of the integrator is integrating the current coming out of the working electrode for a time t_{int} that is determined by the voltage reference $V_{ref \; used}$ by the comparator. The comparator switched its output state when the integrator output gets to V_{ref} level. The main function of the comparator is to produce an output to trigger a one-shot circuitry, which in turns generates a pulse of time period t_{reset} to bring the switches WS1 and WS2 to "off" state. The one-shot stage has a role to generate a pulse width that assures that the switches are completely reset. The one-shot output as shown in the Figure 2-11 also has another function, which is triggering the sequential circuit toggle dynamic flip-flop, which in turns generates a digital signal with frequency value defined by the following equation [20]:

$$f_{out} = \frac{1}{2(t_{int} + t_{reset})} \tag{2.9}$$

This circuit produces digital pulses with the frequency being inversely proportional to the effective capacitance [21] where the sensor and reference capacitance electrode are connected to the readout. The readout circuit translates the analog capacitance difference into a digital output signal. The frequency of the output signal is proportional to the difference of sensor and reference capacitance as well [22].

Simplified equivalent circuit shown in Figure 2-12 can model the biosensor based on capacitance measurement. In general, the model is a capacitance in parallel with a resistance. The superior behavior of the capacitance can be achieved by the excellent capacitor dielectric that has a very large shunt resistance.

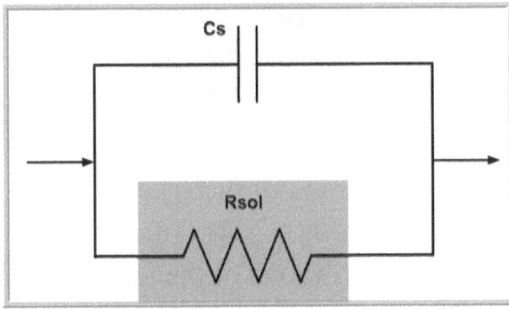

Figure 2-12 IDMA simplified equivalent circuit

As long as the bioreporter sensing concentration of the bacterial pathogen is present in the microfluidic channel, the impedance of the electrolyte (Z) will change. In the light of Ohm's law:

$$I = \frac{V}{Z_T} \qquad (2.10)$$

Where the total impedance Z_T is combined of two parts; real part Z_{Re} the increase of the resistance of the solution and the imaginary part Z_{Im} decrease the double layer capacitance accordingly: given as:

$$Z_T = Z_{Re} + Z_{Im} \qquad (2.11)$$

$Z_{Re} = R_{sol}$ This resistance tends to be vey high $R_{sol} \gg$ so this leads it to be:

$$Z_{Im} = -j\frac{1}{2\pi f C} \qquad (2.12)$$

leading to:

$$I = -2\pi f C \, V_{DD} \qquad (2.13)$$

Where $V_{dd:}$ is the applied voltage.

Therefore, as the capacitance increases due to high concentration, the current flows through sensing the capacitance increase as well. The higher the concentration of the bacterial, the lower the impedance, the more current flow and the higher the frequency occurs. The smaller the amount of the sensing signals of the system is the more sensitive it becomes. This criterion is considered as one of the most important specification of the transducer. The transducer based on capacitance measurements is a smart sensing system for a very low concentration of environmental biological domain.

Consequently, the bioreceptor and the signal-processing circuit play an important role through out the measurement process

2.2.4 Signal and frequency

The SNR ratio of the capacitive biosensors can be defined by the ratio of excitation voltage to the amplifier voltage noise. The theoretical limit of the excitation voltage and a high-impedance amplifier will become corruptive if the amplifier current noise becomes significant. The amplifier current resulting either from very high impedance sensors or from the amplifier input capacitance is superior to sensor capacitance. Therefore, using the CMOS operation amplifier can help significantly in this region due to their lowest noise current [23]. Electronic circuit convertors usually translate capacitance changes into an output signals such as voltage, frequency, or pulse width modulation. In biosensors, systems where the capacitance is in femto or less range than the appropriate electronic convertors should avoid excess of leakage. The applied frequency range must be high enough in order to reduce the impedance of the IDMA as much as it could to avoid coupling with power waveforms and for the entire biosensor frequency response to be sufficient; i.e. 50 kHz. On the other hand, the applied frequency must be reasonably low enough to simplify the electronic design circuit. It is more preferable to use frequency in a range of 100 KHz to get a good tradeoff. Usually the shape of the excitation signal is either square or in a trapezoidal waveform. Square waveforms are more preferable due to their well-controlled bandwidth. The bandwidth is usually set ten times higher than the excitation frequency for accurate measurements. In some cases, a triangle waveform could apply to permit a simpler amplifier implementation using a resistive feedback. However, a sinusoidal signal boasts generally superior accuracy mainly at high frequency applications. Synchronous demodulators are so helpful in biosensors that they are excited with a continuous waveform in order to boost precision and good rejection of noise [24].

2.2.5 Sensitivity

Sensitivity plays an important role in any design particularly in biosensor applications, current or voltage alterations in consequence of an alteration in the gap between the target and the sensing surface. The sensitivity can be readily obtained graphically by plotting the output voltage versus the gap size; in which the slope of the line is the sensitivity. The sensitivity of the biosensor as a transducer to the target as a sensing layer is proportional to the dielectric constant of the biomaterial. Ultimate capacitance biosensor behavior, such as cancer markers, is required to have stable, highly sensitive and reliable sensing surface at the electrode-electrolyte interface [25].

2.3 CMOS Charge Based Capacitance Measurement Circuit

Charge based capacitance measurement method was originally proposed as an accurate technique for the characterization of interconnects capacitance in deep submicron CMOS integrated circuits. Figure 2-13 shows the principle of operation in which two signal pulses V_p and V_n are applied to two pairs of nMOS and pMOS transistors in order to frequently charge and discharge the sensing capacitor C_S and the reference capacitor C_R. The signals V_p and V_n in Figure 2-13 are two non-overlapping signals. The purpose of these non-overlapping waveforms is to ensure that only one of the two transistors in the basic test structure is conducting current [26].

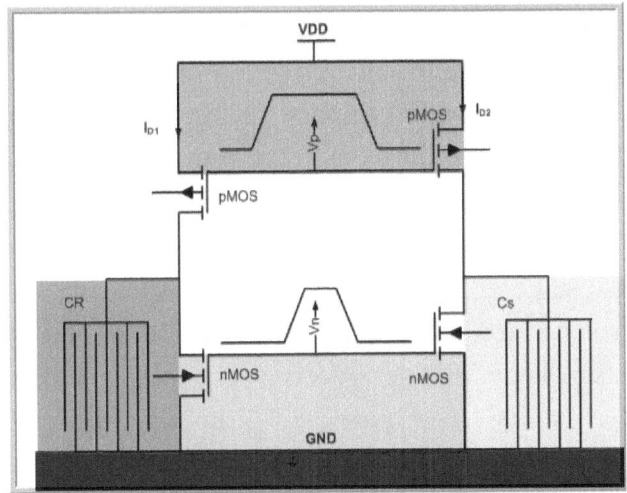

Figure 2-13 Schematic representation of (CBCM).

Thus, the short-circuit current from V_{dd} to ground is eliminated. When the PMOS transistor turns on, it will draw charge from V_{dd} to charge up the target interconnect capacitance. The generated DC currents I_{D1} and I_{D2} can be obtained from the following equations:

$$I_{D1} = V_{DD}.f.C_1 \tag{2.14}$$

$$I_{D2} = V_{DD}.f.C_2 \tag{2.15}$$

Where V_{dd} and f are the power supply voltage and the frequency of clock pulse (V_p and V_n) respectively. Based on this method, the subtraction of charging/discharging currents I_{D1} and I_{D2} measured through high precision DC ammeters is proportional to ΔC [27]:

$$\Delta C = \frac{I_{D1} - I_{D2}}{f.V_{DD}} \tag{2.16}$$

The simplified block diagram of the CBCM circuit shown in Figure 2-14 demonstrates the symmetrical and differential behavior of the circuit, therefore; the initial value of the capacitance does not affect the output voltage. The CBCM circuit has three current mirrors and one voltage follower. The top two current mirrors; (M4-M6 and M5-M7) are used to amplify (A_l) the charging currents in the two branches, where the third current mirror, at the bottom; (M8-M9) is used for transferring the variation of the currents to the next stage to convert them to voltage by using the integrating capacitance.

The last stage is a buffering stage to isolate the circuit from whatever you connect the output of the circuit to has no effect on the circuit itself; voltage follower; receives this voltage to be delivery by the end user for analysis. Figure 2-14 is the schematic of the CBCM circuit. M0-M3 is the CBCM core that can convert the difference ΔC between the two capacitors C_s and C_R into current difference ΔI between two currents I_{D1} and I_{D2}. M4- M9 form current mirrors used to read out and amplify (A_l) ΔI.

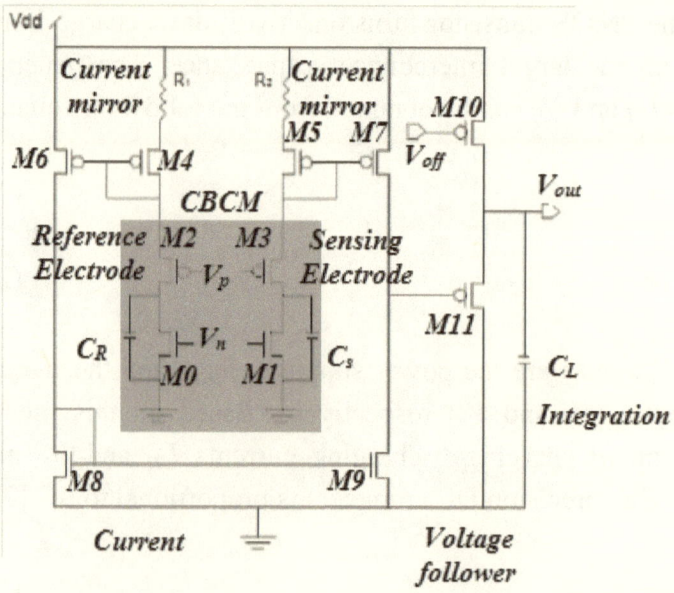

Figure 2-14 CBCM interface circuit topology.

Note that the gain of the current mirror stage is mainly defined by the aspect ratios of M8 and M9. Where M10 and M11 form the voltage follower (A_v) used to drive the load capacitor as a low pass filter. Resistors R_1 and R_2 used to balance the offset caused by the fabrication mismatch and offset caused during the epoxy encapsulation and packaging.

2.4 Experimental Setup and CBCM on MLoC System Validation

In terms of the transduction techniques used, the three main classes of biosensors are optical, electrochemical and magnetic. Almost all current methods of diagnosing tuberculosis (TB) have drawbacks where the level of pathogens in a contaminated sample is often below the detection limits [28], they tend to be either nonspecific or too time-consuming. In most cases of pulmonary TB, diagnosis depends upon culturing the mycobacterium organism, a process requiring 4-8 weeks [29]. To overcome this problem, sample pre-treatment steps and signal amplification strategies are usually required. In CBCM technique, the sensor employs a differential capacitor architecture using the sensing and reference capacitors to achieve improved resolution and higher signal-to-noise ratio. No surface treatment takes place on the reference capacitor and hence it does not experience any capacitance changes with the changes in biological cells concentrations.

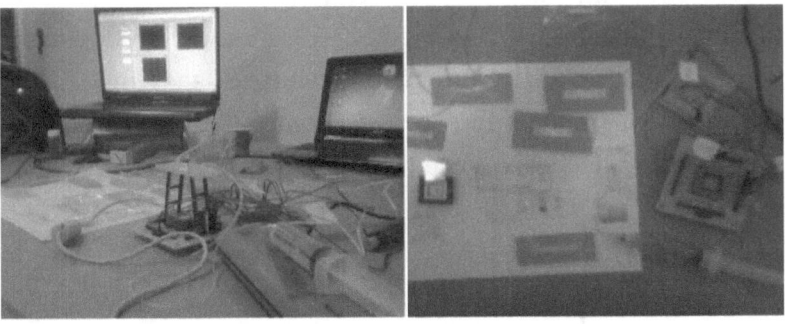

Figure 2-15 The experimental setup for Multibiosensors circuit based on CBCM.

The CMOS CBCM circuit measures the difference of capacitance between the sensing and reference capacitors and provides a proportional voltage output [30][31]. Figure 2-15 shows the measurement principle, interface capacitance determines the frequency of the electrodes charging and discharging transients. A comparator compares the interdigitated microelectrode potential with a reference voltage V_{ref} producing a digital signal at its output. The frequency of the output signal is inversely proportional to capacitance. The integrator accumulates the current signal until its output voltage reaches the threshold of the comparator. Then, the one-shot circuit resets the integrator and triggers the Dynamic Flip-Flop (DFF) [32]. The output frequency of the DFF is the digital representation of the variation of the sensing capacitor. To minimize error and simplify the sensor implementation the output can be read directly without further post processing [33][34].

2.5   CBCM Technique Validation

2.5.1   Simulation Results

In this section, simulation and experimental results of sensing capacitance, interface circuit, interdigitated MMCC capacitance are introduced and discussed. The transient output voltage of the interface circuit Figure 2-13 is simulated using Spectra under Cadence environment for different values of input sensing capacitances (C_s) as shown in Figure 2-14. Figure 2-16 demonstrates the linear relation between output voltage and input sensing capacitances, where the reference capacitance C_R is 500fF. As shown in these figures, this design results in 0.38 mV/fF sensitivity:

$$S = \frac{\Delta V}{\Delta C} = 0.38 \; mV/fF \tag{2.17}$$

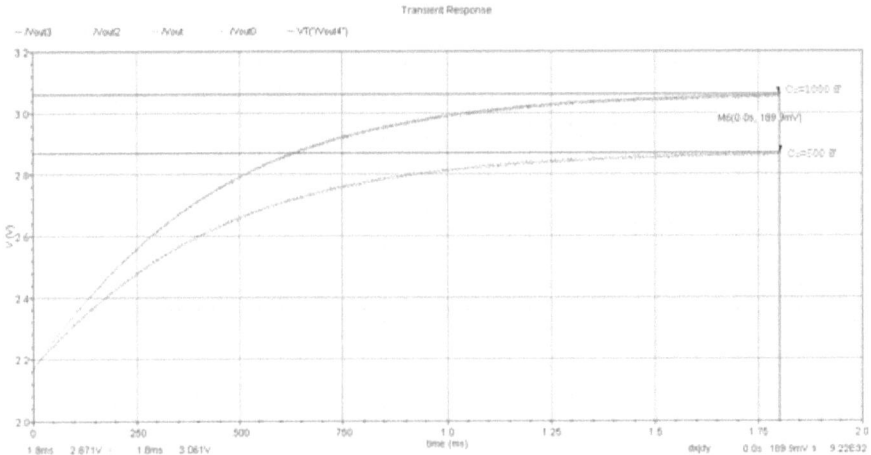

Figure 2-16 Simulation results showing the voltage output of the CBCM circuit.

If there is an unexpected offset in the capacitance value in the CBCM circuit, the value of resistor R can be adjusted to cancel the offset that might occur because of CMOS mismatch issue. Normally; the value of 1/(fC) is much larger than R; hence adjusting the value of the resistance will not have a significant affect on the sensitivity of the circuit. Figure 2-16 shows the Spectra simulation result of the circuit. The output voltage changes from 2.871 V to 3.061 V because of the variation in the capacitance, $\Delta C = 500\ fF$. When similar devices are used on both sides of the CBCM structure, the effects of parasitic capacitances associated with M1-M3 are removed through the capacitance subtraction.

2.5.2   *Capacitance measurements*

Figure 2-17 shows the variation of the capacitance with respect to the frequency. These results are extracted from the experimental setup as shown in Figure 2-15. Figure 2-18 illustrates the capacitance measurements within low frequency.

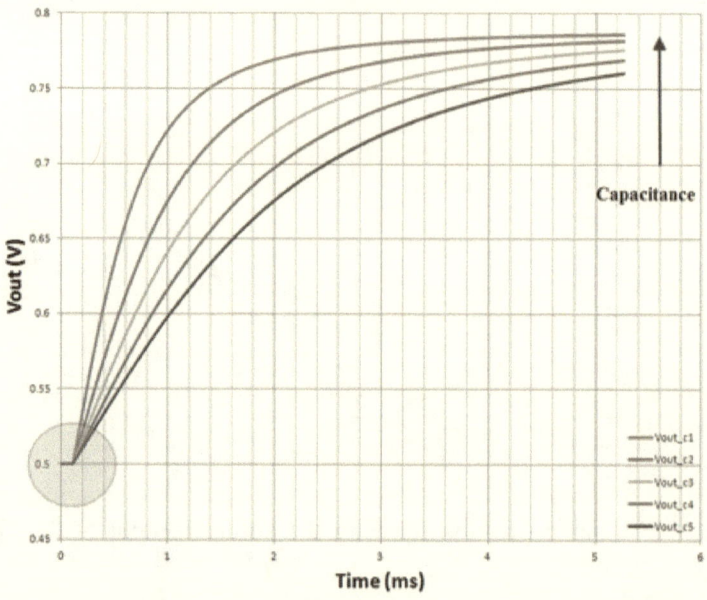

Figure 2-17 The capacitance measurement using CMOS capacitance biosensor.

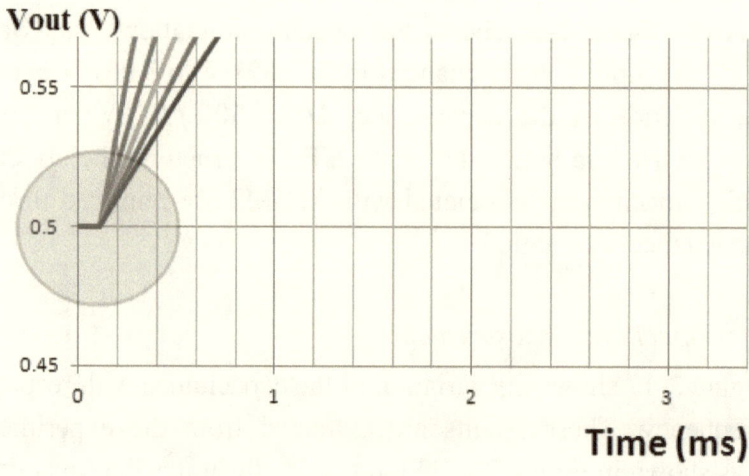

Figure 2-18 The capacitance measurement shows no significant response at low frequency range.

2.5.3 Summary

This part of the book focused on the CMOS capacitive-based biosensor as one part out of the four biosensors implemented at once on the multi-labs-on-single-chip (MLoC) system that was realized through CMOS technology. The CBCM technique on the MLoC system is tested in appropriate conditions and its performance was validated. The system provided a viable alternative to traditional biological analysis systems, which is mostly time consuming. The system employs an interdigitated capacitor structure in the charge based capacitance measurement technique to detect and process capacitance variations in the presence of targeted biological cells. The system provides a rapid, low power, and miniaturized platform that can be used for mass-production. As stated, originality consists of three categories that each includes two components, the use of ideas and tools. The first category consists of old ideas that are implemented using new tools to create the final result. As for the second category, it consists of new ideas invented that are then put to work using old tools. The third and final category under originality includes newly invented ideas and the use of new tools. A fourth aspect of this is the use of old tools and old ideas, which is not considered originality at all. In the light of the definition of originality, the CBCM techniques fill in the first category where the ideas have been previously published since 1984 but the tools used to create the first biosensor out of four in the MLoC-system are CMOSP35, which is one of the most recent technologies. In addition, the reference electrode in this technique is isolated using a special layer made of combinations of CMOSP35 metals, which fill in the third category of originality. Furthermore, the Signal process unit used to avoid the parasitic capacitance that due to the pins and connectors, which makes the biosensors more reliable and sensitive.

2.6 References

[1] James C. Chen, Bruce W. McGaughy, Dennis Sylvester, and Chenming Hu, "An On-Chip, Attofarad Interconnect Charge-Based Capacitance Measurement (CBCM) Technique", IEEE 1996.

[2] L. K. Baxter, "Appendix 1: Capacitive Sensors in Silicon Technology", Capacitive Sensors, Design and Applications, Page(s): 279-285, 2000.

[3] Lion Precision, "Capacitive Sensor Operation and Optimization", 2009.

[4] Dennis Sylvester, James C. Chen, and Chenming Hu, "Investigation of Interconnect Capacitance Characterization Using Charge-Based Capacitance Measurement (CBCM) Technique and Three-Dimensional Simulation", IEEE journal of solid-state circuits, vol. 33, no. 3, pp 449-453, March 1998.

[5] Jeffrey A. Babcock, Scott G. Balster, Angelo Pinto, Christoph Dirnecker, Philipp Steinmann, Reiner Jumpertz, and Badih El-Kareh, "Analog Characteristics of Metal-Insulator-Metal Capacitors Using PECVD Nitride Dielectrics". IEEE electron device letters, vol. 22, no. 5, May 2001.

[6] Bruce W. McGaughy, James C. Chen, Dennis Sylvester, and Chenming Hu, "A Simple Method for On-Chip, Sub-Femto Farad Interconnect Capacitance Measurement", IEEE Electron device letters, vol. 18, no. 1, January 1997.

[7] Kummer, A.M.; Hierlemann, A.; "Configurable electrodes for capacitive-type sensors and chemical sensors", Sensors Journal, IEEE, Volume: 6, Issue: 1, 2006, Page(s): 3-10.

[8] Winncy Y. Du and 2Scott W. Yelich, "Resistive and Capacitive Based Sensing Technologies", Sensors &

Transducers Journal, Vol. 90, Special Issue, April 2008, pp. 100-116.

[9]   Fernandez-Sanchez C, McNeil CJ, Rawson K, Nilsson O., "Disposable noncompetitive immunosensor for free and total prostate-specific antigen based on capacitance measurement", Anal Chem 2004;76:5649-56.

[10]   Gary S. Sayler, Steven Ripp, David Nivens, Michael Simpson, "Bioluminescent Bioreporter Integrated Circuit; Sensing Analytes and Organism with Living Microoranisms", Journal of Environmental Biotechnology, Vol. 1, No. 1, 33-39, 2001.

[11]   Roberto de la Rica, Antonio Baldi, Cesar Fernandez-Sanchez and Hiroshi Matsui, "Selective Detection of Live Pathogens via Surface-Confined Electric Field Perturbation on Interdigitated Silicon Transducers", Anal. Chem., 2009, 81 (10), pp 3830-3835, March 31, 2009.

[12]   Roberto de la Rica, Antonio Baldi, and César Fernández-Sánchez, "Local detection of enzymatic ion generation with polycrystalline silicon interdigitated electrodes and its application to biosensing", Appl. Phys. Lett., Volume, 90, Issue 7, 074102, 2007.

[13]   Roberto de la Rica, César Fernández-Sánchez, Antonio Baldi, "Electric preconcentration and detection of latex beads with interdigitated electrodes", Appl. Phys. Lett. 90, 174104, 2007.

[14]   Roberto de la Rica, César Fernández-Sánchez, Antonio Baldi, "Polysilicon interdigitated electrodes as impedimetric sensors", Electrochemistry Communications, Volume 8, Issue 8, August 2006, Pages 1239-1244.

[15]   R. de la Rica, "New concept for electrical detection of biomolecules", 2007.

[16]   Peter Van Gerwen, Wim Laureyn, Wim Laureys, Guido Huyberechts, Maaike Op De Beeck, Kris Baert, Jan Suls,

Willy Sansen, P. Jacobs, Lou Hermans, Robert Mertens, "Nanoscaled interdigitated electrode arrays for biochemical sensors", Sensors and Actuators B: Chemical, Volume 49, Issues 1-2, Pages 73-80, 25 June 1998.

[17]   Randy Bach, Bob Davis, Rich Laubhan, "Improvements to CBCM (Charge-Based Capacitance Measurement) for Deep Submicron CMOS Technology", Proceedings of the 7th International Symposium on Quality Electronic Design, IEEE, 2006.

[18]   Eric K. Bolton, Gary S. Sayler, David E. Nivens, James M. Rochelle, Steven Ripp, Michael L. Simpson, "Integrated CMOS photodetectors and signal processing for very low-level chemical sensing with the bioluminescent bioreporter integrated circuit", Sensors and Actuators B: Chemical, Volume 85, Issues 1-2, Pages 179-185, 20 June 2002.

[19]   Michael L. Simpson, Gary S. Sayler, James T. Fleming, Bruce Applegate, "Whole-cell biocomputing", Trends in Biotechnology, Volume 19, Issue 8, Pages 317-323, 1 August 2001.

[20]   R. Vijayaraghavan, S.K. Islam, M. Zhang, S. Ripp, S. Caylor, Nora D. Bull, S. Moser, S.C. Terry, B.J. Blalock, G.S. Sayler, "A bioreporter bioluminescent integrated circuit for very low-level chemical sensing in both gas and liquid environments", Sensors and Actuators B: Chemical, Volume 123, Issue 2, Pages 922-928, 21 May 2007.

[21]   Michael S.-C. Lu, Yi-Chung Chen, Dong-Che Li, and Po-Chiun Huang, "CMOS capacitive sensors for ultrasensitive dopamine detection".

[22]   R. Singh, R. Genov, R. Kotamraju, B. Mazhari, "Multi-Step Binary-Weighted Capacitive Digital-to-Analog Converter Architecture," IEEE Midwest Symposium on Circuits and Systems (MWSCAS'08), Knoxville, Tennessee, Aug. 10-13, 2008.

[23] Ebrahim Ghafar-Zadeh, Mohamad Sawan, Daniel Therriault, "CMOS based capacitive sensor laboratory-on-chip: a multidisciplinary approach", Analog Integr Circ Sig Process, 59:1-12. 2009.

[24] Iwan Evans, Trevor York, "Microelectronic capacitance transducer for particle detection", Sensors Journal, IEEE, Volume: 4, Issue: 3, Page(s): 364-372, June 2004.

[25] Sandro Carrara, Vijayender Bhalla, Claudio Stagni, Luca Benini, Anna Ferretti, Francesco Valle, Andrea Gallotta, Bruno Riccò, Bruno Samorì, "Label-free cancer markers detection by capacitance biochip", Sensors and Actuators B: Chemical, Volume 136, Issue 1, 2 February 2009, Pages 163-172.

[26] Somashekar Bangalore Prakash, Pamela, Abshire, Mario Urdaneta, Elisabeth Smela, "A CMOS Capacitance Sensor for Cell Adhesion Characterization".

[27] Sowlati, T. Vathulya, V. Leenaerts, D., "High density capacitance structures in submicron CMOS for low power RF applications", ISLPED '01. August 6-7, pp. 243-246, 2001.

[28] Shi-Wei Wang and M. S.-C. Lu, "CMOS Capacitive Sensors with Sub-um Microelectrodes for Biosensing Applications," to appear in IEEE Sensors Journal, 2010.

[29] M.-H. Chen and M. S.-C. Lu, "Design and characterization of an air-coupled capacitive ultrasonic sensor fabricated in a CMOS process," J. Micromech. and Microeng., vol. 18, 2008.

[30] Brian Ward, Jim Bordelon, Scott Prior, Ben Tranchina, and Jiann Liu, "Test Structure and Method for Capacitance Extraction in Multi-Conductor Systems", Proc. IEEE 2001 Int. Conference on Microelectronic Test Structures, Vol. 14, March 2001.

[31] Zhenqiu Ning, Henri-Xavier Delecourt, Luc De Schepper, Renaud Gillon, "Precise Analogue Characterization of MIM

Capacitors Using an Improved Charge-Based Capacitance Measurement (CBCM) Technique", Proceedings of ESSDERC, Grenoble, France, 2005.

[32]   R. Jacob Baker, Harry W. Li, David E. Boyce, "CMOS Circuit Design, Layout, and Simulation", pp433, 1998, 2ed. New York: Wiley-IEEE Press, 2008

[33]   Jay Rajagopalan, Haris Basit, "Optimization of Metal-Metal Comb-Capacitors for RF Applications" RF Products Group National Semiconductor Corporation Federal, OEA International Inc.

[34]   Martin J. Brophy, Alfredo Torrejon, Shawn Petersen, Kamal Avala, and Li Liu, "MIM's the Word-Capacitors for Fun and Profit", TriQuint Semiconductor.

Chapter 3 - CMOS single-chip Optical Biosensors

3.1   Introduction

There is widespread demand for a low-cost, highly miniaturized, rapid, selective and highly sensitive detection method for low-abundance detection in biological and biomedicine applications such as bacteria and cancer markers. The detection of weakly expressed proteins and protein complexes in biological samples down to single-molecule level represents a major challenge for scientists, due to the difficulty to achieve an acceptable level of signal-to-noise ratio. In addition, analysis of low abundance analysts can take several hours to days to give accurate results, and require bulky, expensive equipment. In this work, a highly miniaturized and integrated Multilabs-on-a-single-chip system has developed. The system comprises a fluorescence CMOS reader, a microfluidic channel, an analyte manipulation/concentration system and a novel amplification strategy for the binding event signal in the microfluidic system. A high sensitive phototransistor built as 32 by 32 arrays has been developed for biosensor detection using CMOSP35 technology. A high-gain emitter inversion layer in VPNP emerges in CMOS technology to design a phototransistor array, to enhance the electrical characteristics of the CMOS analogue; as a result, the current gain β is improved. In such technology, diffused source/drain junctions are used as merged VPNP emitters.

In this chapter, we use nanosensors based on optical biosensors; fluorescence sensing mechanisms that has been introduced and discussed in [1]. These optical sensors usually employ bacteriophage or phageorganisms as recognition elements to detect bacteria such as E-Coli. Fluorescence spectroscopy can apply to a wide range of problems in the chemical and biological sciences. The measurements can provide information on a wide range of molecular processes, including the interactions of solvent molecules with fluorophores, rotational diffusion of biomolecules, binding interactions, conformational changes, and distances between sites on biomolecules. Advances in technology for cellular imaging and single-molecule detection are expanding the usefulness of fluorescence. These advances in fluorescence technology have short response time, are simple to implement, and they are standoff detection [2]. Moreover, the cost and complexity are greatly reduced making these sensors commercially competitive. Fluorescence spectroscopy will continue to contribute to rapid advances in biology, biotechnology, medical diagnostics, DNA sequencing, forensics, genetic analysis and nanotechnology [3]. Fluorescence detection is highly sensitive, and there is no longer the need for the expensive and complex radioactive tracers for most biochemical measurements. There has been dramatic growth in the use of fluorescence for cellular and molecular imaging. Fluorescence imaging can reveal the localization and measurements of intracellular molecules, sometimes at the level of single-molecule detection.

Typically, fluorescence based sensors excite optically active recognition elements that are selective to particular media (i.e. LB). Emission from the bacteriophage, at wavelengths is longer than the excitation wavelength, and it is monitored. It also provides information regarding the concentration of multiple bacteria or viruses in real-time. Thus, in this technique, it is important to immobilize the bacteriophage at the sensor surface and maximize the contact surface area to maximize the interaction of the media with the recognition element during the sensor operation. A phageorganisms (phage) is a type of virus that infects bacteria.

This work is capable to detect and act as an atto-molar cancer markers concentration as long as these markers are based on CMOS optical biosensor and are used for biological and life science applications detection.

3.2 CMOS Phototransistor technique

The CMOS phototransistor, that is a highly photosensitive sensor, is necessary for the system because the biosensor area is small. Therefore, the phototransistor has been developed using the CMOSP35 process. The Emitter is a p diffusion layer in an n-well. Stripe shape is used to reduce the parasitic capacitance of the phototransistor. The P-type substrate acts as a collector. The structure forms photodiode when the n-well is connected to the supply voltage. On the other hand, the phototransistor is formed when the potential of n-well is floating. The factor of β amplifies the photocurrent between the n-well to the p-type substrate. To enhance the electrical characteristics of the CMOS analogue or the digital circuits, IC designers often employ merged vertical bipolar transistors (VPNP) coexisting on the same substrate as CMOS [9]. In such 'pseudo-BiCMOS' technology, diffused source/drain junctions are commonly used as merged VPNP emitters. Theoretically, there are two main factors, which limit the static current gain β: the first factor is a low bipolar injection efficiency of source/drain P^+ emitters; the second factor is the enhanced parasitic sidewall injection of $P+$ emitters in a compensated N-well base surface.

This chapter introduces the design and implementation of an optical biosensor system with improved and tunable detection sensitivity. The circuit is implemented using CMOS technology along with VPNP technology. The IC consists of high-gain phototransistors in a form of a 32 by 32 array. Figure 3-1 shows the architecture of this design. The integrated circuit separates the data by selecting the arbitrary light receiving element depending on the status of light source. In order to avoid the light receiving element from being insensitive due to the shrinkage in its surface area, the phototransistor that is more sensitive than photodiode was adopted as the light receiving element with the standard CMOSP35 technology.

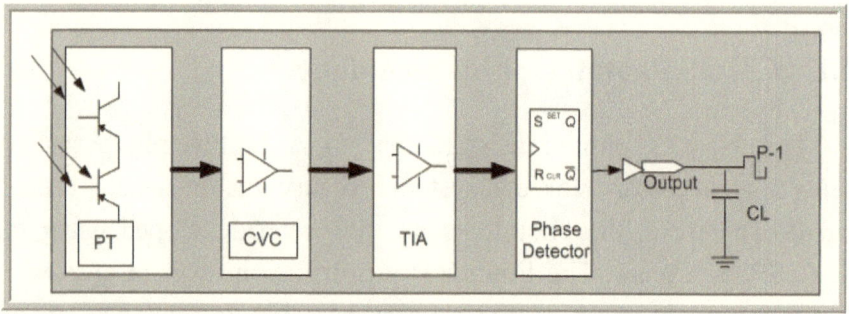

Figure 3-1   CMOS Detection and Signal-Processing Circuit.

In addition, the trans-impedance amplifier (TIA) was adopted. Its sensitivity and response frequency were optimized according to the carrier frequency of visible light ID system and the characteristic of phototransistor. Each light receiving element is arbitrarily selectable with the external signal and capable of increasing the sensitivity by selecting more than one light receiving the element simultaneously [10]. The structure of the phototransistor pixel is similar to a bipolar junction transistor and is formed by p-active (emitter)/n-well (base)/p-substrate (collector). This phototransistor structure was selected because of its highest responsivity (electrical current output/optical power input) of the photodetectors available in the standard CMOS process and particularly in the visible region of the electromagnetic spectrum. Phototransistors in a form of 32 by 32 arrays have been developed as a fluorometric biosensor system using the single-chip CMOS detection and processing unit, and the sensor system determines analyte concentrations. An external excitation source has been used through out this work; red laser 630-680 nm; or blue laser 473 nm, and the fluorescence is detected by the optical chip using a phototransistor that is 32 x 32 array. The optical chip also includes a current mirror, a current-to-voltage converter, an amplifier, a band-pass filter, and a phase detector. The optical chip output is a DC voltage that corresponds to the detected fluorescence phase shift. The main targeted design goals for this biosensor system are stability, reproducibility, analytical reliability, and fast response to changes. The low cost, low power and miniaturization are part of the design requirements. Regulated Cascade (RGC)-type circuit as trans-impedance amplification (TIA) converts the current signal from the phototransistor into the voltage. A trans-impedance amplifier circuit is adapted to achieve high gain, low noise and wide band characteristics. The complete schematic including the bias circuit is shown in Figure 3-2 [32]. The circuit was fabricated using CMOSP35 technology. The conversion gain of the TIA depends on its self-resistance. Therefore, the phototransistor made of CMOSP35 process is more sensitive to the frequency characteristic due to a negative impact of parasitic capacitance, compared to the Positive-Intrinsic-Negative (PIN) photodiode. The IC essentially consists of four blocks; the phototransistor array; the current to voltage converter; the amplifier block; and the phase detector as demonstrated in Figure 3-1. The phototransistor array forms the high-sensitivity phototransistors that are capable to convert the imposed optical signals into electrical current signals and send the signals to an operational amplifier (op-amp) based circuit that acts as a current-to-voltage converter.

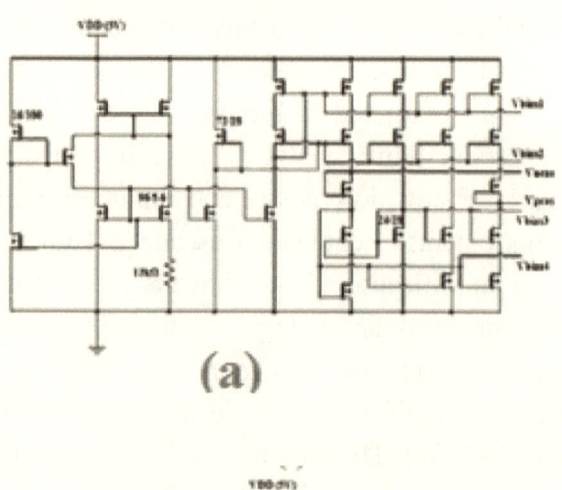

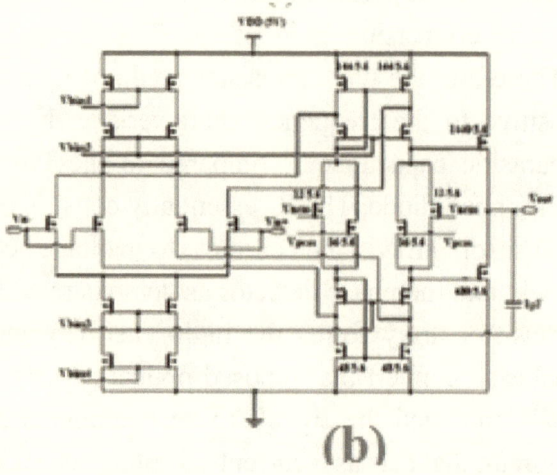

Figure 3-2 (a) Schematic of the bias generator circuit for rail-to-rail folded-cascade op-amp used in CVC and TIA. (b) Schematic of the folded-cascade and output stages of the op-amp.

Another operational amplifier based circuit amplifies the following voltage signals and then the signal is sent to a XNOR based phase detector. The nonlinear phase detector is an XNOR type detector that provides a dc voltage proportional to the phase shift between the detected optical signal and a fixed reference sinusoidal signal produced by a standard function generator [32].

66

3.3   VPNP phototransistor operation

Phototransistors made of silicon act as photosensors and respond to the entire visible radiation range. The Phototransistor is a photodiode with amplification. The Phototransistor light sensor has its collector-base PN-junction reverse biased exposing it to the radiant light source. In essence, a phototransistor can be a bipolar transistor either PNP or NPN configuration whose outer casing is either transparent or has a clear lens to focus the light onto the base junction for increased sensitivity. Phototransistors consist mainly of a bipolar NPN transistor with its large base region electrically unconnected, although some phototransistors allow a base connection to control the sensitivity, which uses photons of light to generate a base current, which in turn causes a current to flow from the collector to the emitter. In fact, the operation of a phototransistor is based on the biasing arrangement and light frequency. Phototransistor in its two types; NPN and PNP, mainly operates in two modes either an active mode or a switch mode. In the active mode, the operation of the phototransistor produces a response proportional to the incident light that is received by the exposed part up to a certain light level. At the time the amount of light exceeds that level, the phototransistor turns out to be saturated and the output will not boost neither affect anything additional in the light level. In the switch mode, the operation of the phototransistor will be either Off-state or On-state in response to the light.

The VPNP phototransistor in the homo-junction planar structure as shown in Figure 3-3 is composed of two back-to-back diodes, PN and NP as shown in Figure 3-4. The biasing arrangement plays a key role in the photosensor's mechanism [11]. In forward biased configuration, the junction NP is the collector-base diode of the bipolar transistor. In this case, the increased current through the junctions due to incident light will be negligible. In contrast, in the reverse biased NP configuration, the boost in current flow will be significant and will be responsible for the light intensity.

Dr. Abdullah Tashtoush

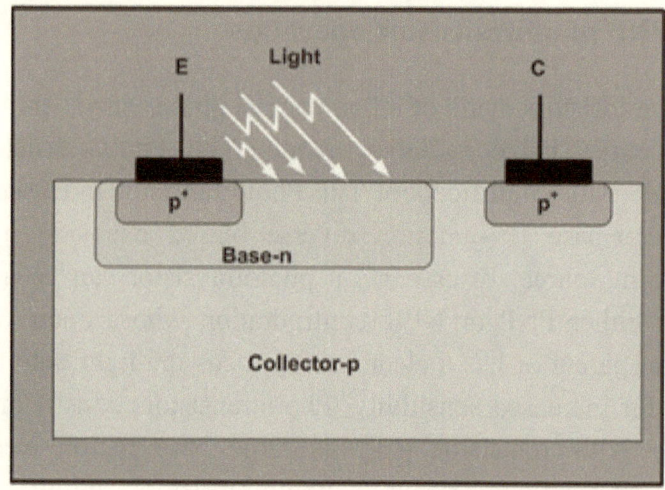

Figure 3-3   PNP phototransistor homo-junction planar structure.

The optimum conversion and hence sensitivity can be accomplished by making the emitter contact offset within the phototransistor structure.

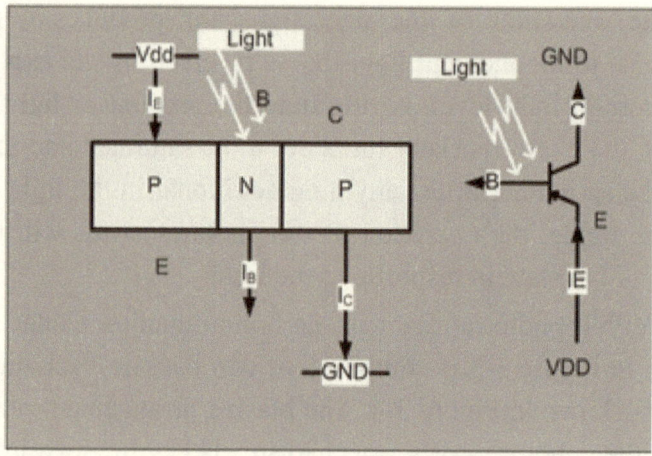

Figure 3-4   The PNP phototransistor operation.

This technique ensures that the maximum amount of incident light gets in touch with the active region within the phototransistor structure. For this reason, the PNP phototransistors are operated in active mode. This means that the junction emitter-based is forward biased and the collector-base junction is reverse biased. In such application, where the light is part of the operation, the base connection is floating; in fact, the light-induced current effectively replaces the base current. The gate (G) terminal would only be used to bias the phototransistor with the intention that additional collector current was flowing and this would mask any current flowing because of the light intensity achievement.

The base of the phototransistor is left as an open terminal, where the gate can be used to bias the device to a constant DC level. Typically, the characteristics of the transistors change due to the base current that leads to a change in the collector current, significantly lead ing to enhance the current gain β. The mechanism of the operational phototransistor heavily depends on the biasing arrangement. This could be simplified by making the collector of a p-n-p transistor negative with respect to the emitter. Hole-electron pairs will be generated thanks to the light penetration into the base region of the phototransistor. For this reason, the collector-base junction should be reverse bias to have the most adequate and readable result from the phototransistor operation. The hole-electron pairs move under the influence of the electric field and provide the base current, causing electrons to be injected into the emitter [12]. The value of β depends on the base current as well, while there is a risk that the junction capacitance C_j becomes large due to the Miller effect and the response frequency gets lower [13].

The Miller effect electronically refers to the increase in the equivalent input capacitance of an inverting voltage amplifier that is caused by the amplification of capacitance between the input and output of the electrical component. The input capacitance is equal to "$C_M = C(1 - A_V)$" where A_v is the gain of the amplifier and C is the feedback capacitance. The ideal voltage amplifier of gain A_v with an impedance Z is connected between its input and output nodes where the input resistance tends to be very high; "$R \rightarrow \infty$" so the input impedance will be equivalent to the input capacitance; "$Z_{in} = \frac{1}{j\omega C}$". The output voltage of the ideal circuitry is given by; "$V_o = A_v V_i$" and the input current is; "$I_i = \frac{V_i - V_o}{Z}$", this leads to an input impedance described as; "$Z_{in} = \frac{1}{j\omega C(1 - A_v)} = \frac{1}{j\omega C_M}$" where C_M is the Miller capacitance.

3.4   VPNP phototransistor Structure and CMOS technology

A lot of effort was devoted to enhance the behavior of the detecting circuit. The result of that is the generation of the vertical bipolar phototransistor integrated in CMOS technology employing the Inversion Emitter concept [14]. The inversion emitter substantially increases current gain, particularly at low current levels, which leads to a high output photocurrents. In addition, the external gate voltage can control current gain and photocurrent magnitude.

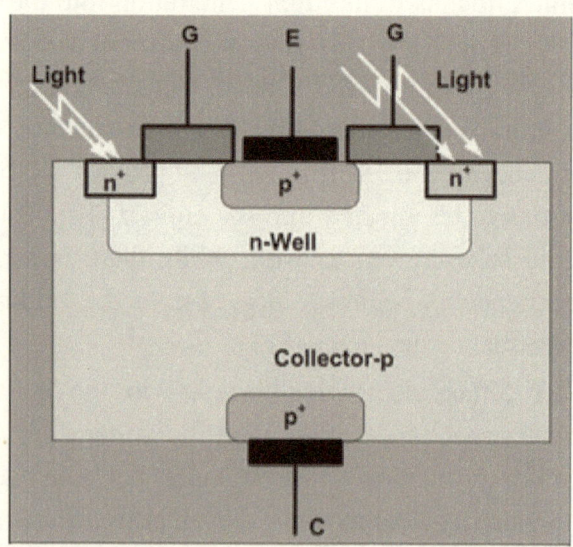

Figure 3-5   Schematic diagram of VPNP phototransistor structure.

By using this concept in the biosensor, the current gain can be boosted further by the current gain of the photodetector structure based on a bipolar transistor. Using MOS transistors, the bipolar transistors could be switched between the "ON" and "OFF" states. Figure 3-5 shows the VPNP phototransistor structure. The inversion emitter improves the overall factor β of VPNP for two reasons: first, the inversion emitter efficiency is inherently improved. Second, the presence of MOS inversion layer decreases the total base current by eliminating minority-carrier surface-recombination in the channel area. The net effect is a substantial improvement of factor β at low current levels in spite of the large VPNP area, where the total collector current for the most part is due to the carriers' photo generated in the base-collector junction contribution which is given by $I_C = \beta I_B$ [15]. The structure of the phototransistor pixel using the vertical phototransistor (VPNP) can produce currents that are several times larger compared to a comparable sized photodiode. The property of the optical biosensor prototype is as following:

1. The IC consists of a high-gain phototransistors 32 by 32 array.
2. The structure of the phototransistor pixel is similar to a bipolar junction transistor and is formed by the p-active (emitter)/n-well (base)/p-substrate (collector).
3. The phototransistor has one of the highest responsivity (electrical current output/optical power input) of the photodetectors available in the standard CMOS process and particularly in the visible region of the electromagnetic spectrum.
4. The vertical phototransistor (VPNP) can produce currents that are several times larger compared to a comparable sized photodiode.

3.4.1   Biosensors Responsivity and Quantum Efficiency

In general, the behavior of the optical transducer can be characterized for a given light source illumination level. The output of a phototransistor can be defined by the area of the exposed collector-base junction and the factor β. The collector-base junction of the phototransistor works like a photodiode through generating a photocurrent, which is fed into the base of the transistor section. Thus, like the case for a photodiode, doubling the size of the base region doubles the amount of the generated base photocurrent. The DC current gain inherent to the transistor amplifies this photocurrent (I_P). For the case where no external base-drive current is applied, the collector current defines as follow:

$$I_C = \beta(I_P) \tag{3.1}$$

Where β is the DC current gain and I_P is the photocurrent. Similar to signal transistors, β varies with base drive, bias voltage and temperature. At low light intensity; β increases with increasing light (or base drive) until a peak is reached. As the light level is further increased, the gain of the phototransistor starts to decrease [16]. The responsivity of a silicon photodiode is a measure of the sensitivity to light, and it defines as the ratio of the photocurrent I_P to the incident light power P at a given wavelength:

$$\mathcal{R} = \frac{I_P}{P_{in}} \tag{3.2}$$

In other words, it is a measure of the effectiveness of the conversion of the light power into electrical current. It varies with the wavelength of the incident light, the applied reverse bias and temperature as shown in Figure 3-6. Quantum efficiency is defined as the fraction of the incident photons that contribute to photocurrent. It relates to responsivity by:

$$\eta = \mathcal{R}\,\frac{hc}{\lambda q} = 1243\,\frac{\mathcal{R}}{\lambda}\,\left(\frac{\mu W}{A}\right) \tag{3.3}$$

Where h is called the Planck constant and is equal to 6.63×10^{-34} J-s, c is the speed of light and is equal to 3×10^8 m/s, q is the electron charge and equals to 1.6×10^{-19} C, $(\mathcal{R})$ is the responsivity in (A/W) and λ is the wavelength in nanometer (nm).

Responsivity $(\mathcal{R})$ in optical biosensors refer to its sensitivity. The quantity of the responsivity is the amount of induced photocurrent generated by the photodetector in response to the external light excitation. The sensitivity for a particular photodetector structure varies as a function of wavelength; the typical values of responsivity for silicon are 0.6 A/W at 900 nm.

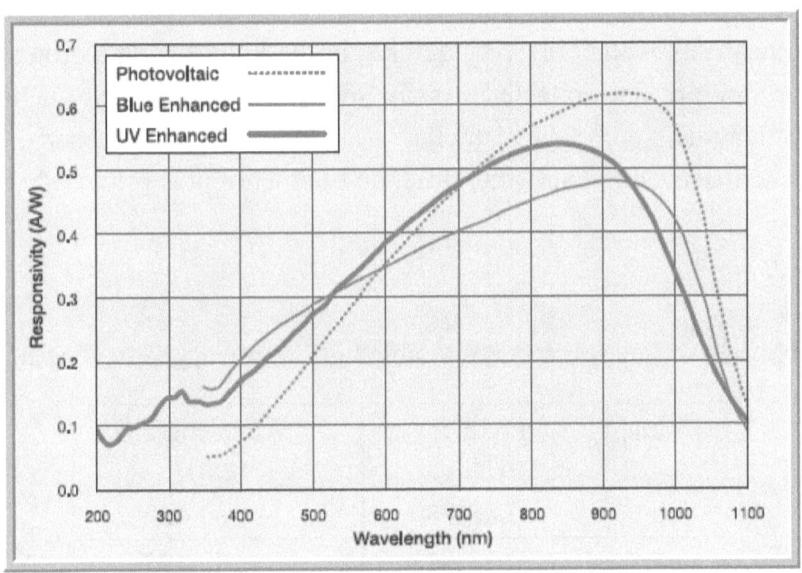

Figure 3-6   Responsivity $(\mathcal{R})$ in optical biosensors varies with the wavelength of the incident light.

Quantum efficiency is well-known as the fraction of the incident photons that contribute to photocurrent meaning that the percentage of collected carriers that are converted into electrical current [17]. The mechanism of generation photocurrent (I_P) in the photodetector lies on the absorption of the photon in the exposed area leading to generate an electron-hole pair. Consequently, one of the pair of free charge carriers are capable to reach the p-n junction thus the carrier is collected and it generates a current. Otherwise, the carrier is vanished in the exposed area by filling an orbital atom meaning that the recombination process leads to no photocurrent to generate. Quantum efficiency relates to responsivity by:

$$\eta = \mathcal{R}\,\frac{hc}{\lambda q} = 1243\,\frac{\mathcal{R}}{\lambda}\,(\frac{nW}{A}) \qquad (3.4)$$

The responsivity "$\mathcal{R}$" of the photodetector is a function of quantum efficiency; "η". Where at short wavelengths; "λ", η is low, since absorption occurs very close to the surface and the induced photocarriers recombine very quickly in the high doping region (N^+) thus they are not collected. As for the quantum efficiency at long wavelengths, the layer thickness is too tiny to absorb the photocarriers completely therefore, no photocurrent is produced:

$$\mathcal{R} = \frac{\eta q}{h\nu} \qquad (3.5)$$

Table 3.1   The spectrum of visible light frequency/wavelength.

Color	Frequency (THz)	Wavelength (λ) (nm)
Violet	668-789	380-450
Blue	631-668	450-475
Cyan	606-630	476-495
Green	526-606	495-570
Yellow	508-526	570-590
Orange	484-508	590-620
Red	400-484	620-750

Where: q is the elementary charge, h is the Planck's constant, ν is the radiation frequency, η(eta) is the quantum efficiency;

$$R = \frac{\eta q}{h\nu} = \frac{\eta q \lambda}{hc} \qquad (3.6)$$

In addition, R is proportional to the voltage generated at the photodetector. Therefore, I_P is given by the following equation:

$$I_P = RP_o = \frac{\eta q}{h\nu}P_o = \frac{\eta q \lambda}{hc}P_o = \frac{\eta \lambda}{1243 \times 10^{-9}}P_o \qquad (3.7)$$

Where: I_P is the average photocurrent generated by a steady-state average optical power P_o incident on the photodetector. The VPNP transistor is designed using CMOSP35 TSMC technology. The dimensions of the transistor are as shown in Figure 3-7. The area of the VPNP transistor is the emitter area 100 μm² (10 μm by 10μm) and the base area is 784 μm² (28μm by 28μm).

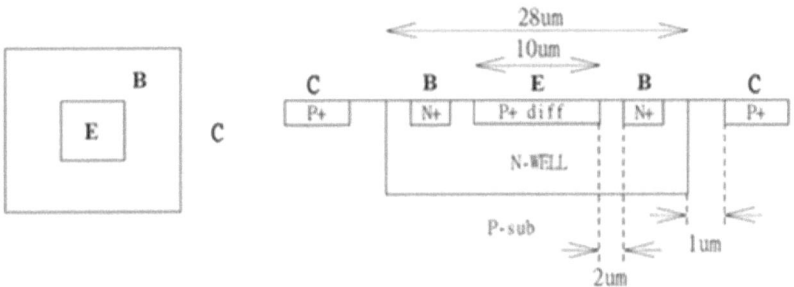

Figure 3-7   The structure of the VPNP transistor as given by CMC.

3.4.2   Phototransistor 32x32 array characteristics

The integration characteristics of the phototransistor can be determined through measuring the time to integrate 1V at different light intensities.

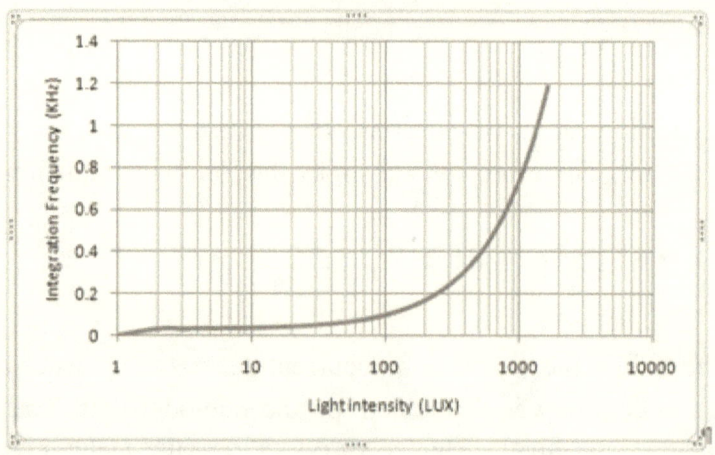

Figure 3-8   Integration frequency vs. light intensity L_i.

The phototransistor at certain light intensities has a linear relationship between the integration frequency and the light intensity (L_i) as shown in Figure 3-8. The light intensities are measured in lumens per square meter (lm/m^2), or *lux* (lx). The current drawn by the phototransistor corresponding to the light intensity can be calculated using the equation of the linear model that measures the relationship between integration frequency and intensity; Eq. (3.9) for a given voltage; 1V and "C_{pt}" is the parasitic capacitance existing in the phototransistor; $C_{pt} = 300\ fF$, as shown in Figure 3-9. The relationship between the current drawn by the phototransistor (I_p) and the light intensity is given by Eq.(3.10) [18]:

$$I_p = \frac{C_{pt}V_{pixel}}{T_{int}} \tag{3.8}$$

$$\frac{1}{T_{int}} = 0.7\ L_i + 32 \tag{3.9}$$

Substitute Eq. (3.9) in Eq.(3.8) which leads to:

$$I_p = C_{pt}V_{pixel}(0.7\ L_i + 32) \tag{3.10}$$

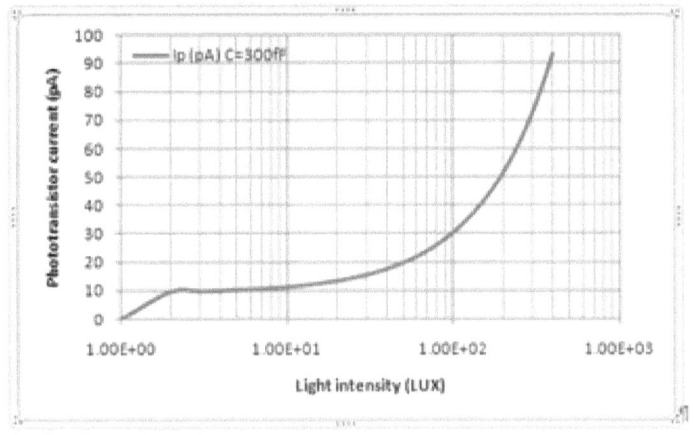

Figure 3-9   The phototransistor current at $C_{pt} = 300\ fF$ and 1 V.

For a given voltage; 1V and C_{pt} is the parasitic capacitance existing in the phototransistor; $C_{pt} = 300\ fF$, the final form of the current I_p is defined as follows:

$$I_p = C_{pt}V_{pixel}((0.7\ L_i) + 32 \times CV = 0.7C_{pt}V_{pixel}(L_i + I_D$$
$$I_p = (2.1 \times 10^{-13}) \cdot L_i + 9.6 \times 10^{-12}$$

Where I_D is the dark current and L_i is the light intensity. I_D is equal to 9.6 pA within the range of the light influence on the silicon as shown in Figure 3-10. The signal-to-noise ratio is figured out by taking the mean swing of each pixel at near saturation and dividing it by the mean of the standard deviation of each pixel.

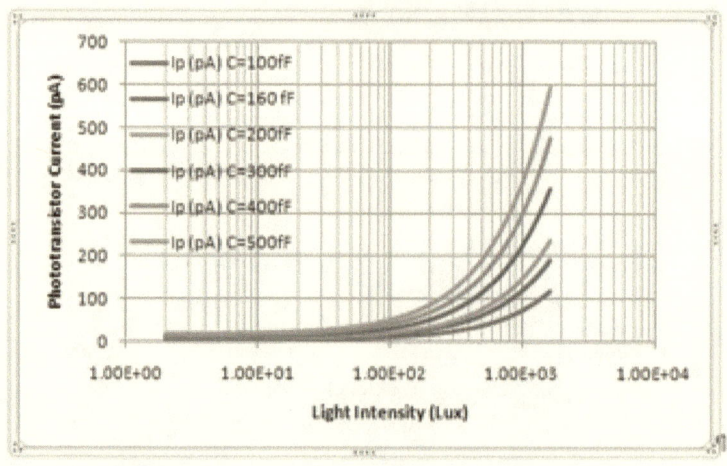

Figure 3-10 Phototransistor current versus light intensity.

The phototransistor reaches saturation level at L_i = 256 *lux*, after T_{in} = 25 μs; so Eq.(3.10) leads to I_P = 63.36 *pA*, thus; from Eq.(3.8) the saturation voltage determined leads to V_{sat} = 5.28 *V*. The standard deviation determined in the dark current I_D = 9.6 *pA* for a short integration time; T_{in} = 10 μs, using Eq. (3.8) leading to:

$$V_{pixel} = \frac{T_{int} \times I_D}{C_{pt}} = \frac{10 \times 10^{-6} \times 9.6 \times 10^{-12}}{300 \times 10^{-15}} = 0.32\ V$$

Hence, SNR = $SNR = \frac{V_{Sat}}{V_{STD}} = \frac{5.28}{0.32} = 16.5$ → 24.30 dB.

Table 3.2   VPNP phototransistor specification

Technology	CMOSP35
Array Size	32 by 32 array
Total Size	1210.8 μm x 1318.4 μm
Pixel Size	40.20 μm x 41.775 μm
Power Consumption	300 μW (@ 3.3V)
Dark Current	9.6 pA

3.4.3   Dark Current (ID)

Most of the characteristics of the phototransistor are similar to the characteristics of a conventional bipolar transistor form. The only exception is the base current replaced by the different levels of light intensity. Usually at a steady state condition where no external potential is applied (i.e. light) to the phototransistor, the operation refers to a tiny amount of current that flows in the structure named the dark current (I_D). Figure 3-11 shows that the dark current (I_D) corresponds to the tiny number of carriers that are attracted to the emitter. This amount of current is, in turns, also subject to the amplification by means of the transistor inherent gain. Therefore, phototransistors are tested to dark current limits, which range from 4.0 *pA* to 80 *pA* with respect to the capacitance range from 10 *fF* to 500 *fF* respectively as shown in Figure 3-12. In order to achieve a certain level of performance by reaching the optimum conversion, the emitter contact is often offset within the phototransistor structure. Achieving that guarantees the maximum amount of incident light that gets in touch with the active region within the phototransistor [19].

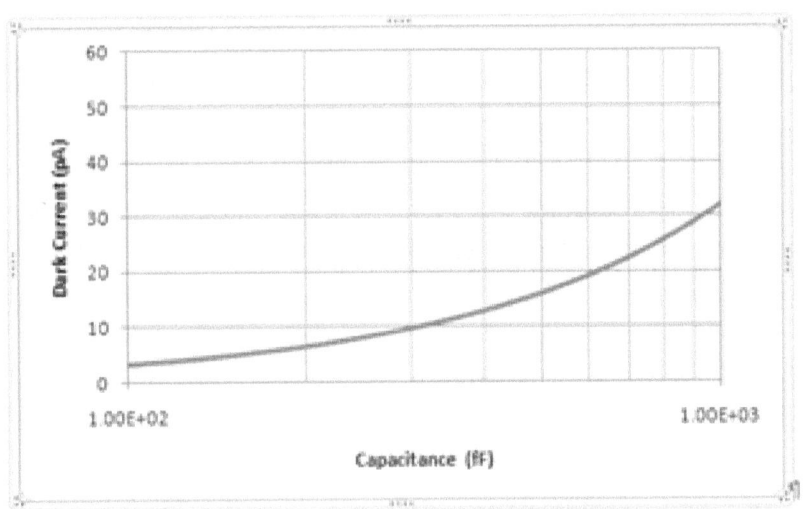

Figure 3-11 Dark current vs. the capacitance.

The dark current is a function of the applied voltage in the basis of the regular transistor operation as shown in Figure 3-13, but this is not the case for the phototransistor structure as long the base terminal is not connect and replaced by the light incident intensity.

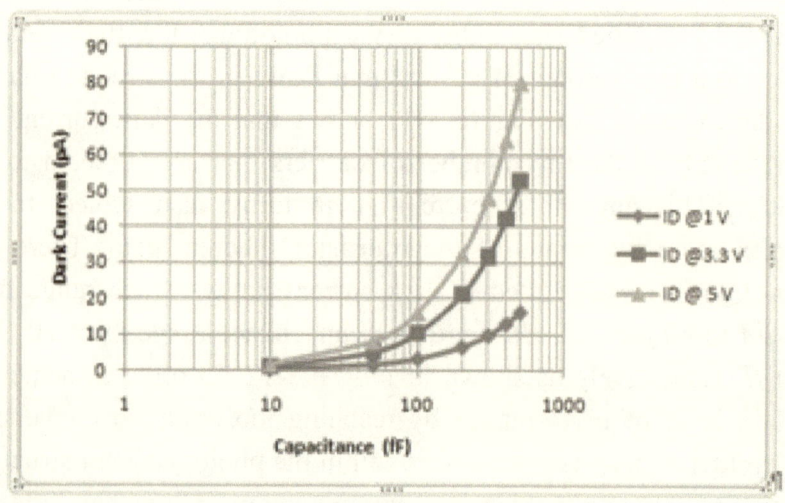

Figure 3-12 The dark current depends on the capacitance.

The mechanism of the dark current that is drawn by the phototransistor corresponds to the light intensity that is acquired when no light is present and a voltage is applied from the collector to the emitter (V_{CE}). For that reason, a certain amount of current will flow. The dark current (I_D) is a leakage current and it can be determined by multiplying the collector-base junction current and the DC current gain β of the transistor. The dark current is a function of the value of the applied voltage V_{CE}. It is also a function to the ambient temperature, where it is directly proportional to it. Therefore, it is usually specified at 25°C. The dark current is considered as a drawback to the phototransistor operation where its presence prevents the device to reach digitally the full ON/OFF states.

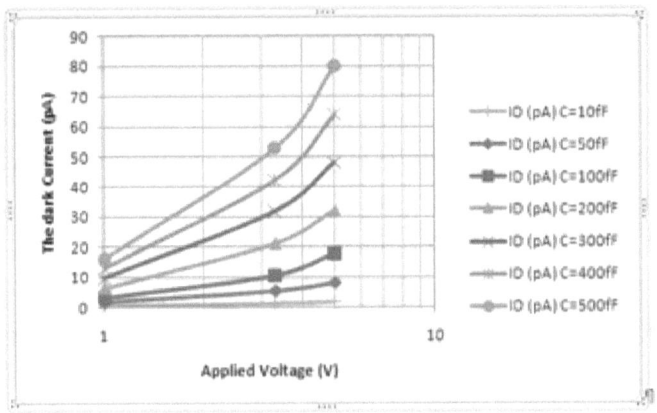

Figure 3-13 The dark current depends on applied voltage.

On the other hand; the dark current offers advantages for the device under test (DUT) at a given collector-emitter test voltage by considering the maximum collector current that is allowed to flow.

3.4.4 Power consumption

One more important phototransistor characteristics is the power consumption. The power consumption can be calculated by observing how much current the biosensor was drawing through the power supply voltage; V_{dd} =3.3 V. The current flow through the phototransistor array and the operational amplifier is measured by a general-purpose multimeter; Keithley 2400. Nevertheless, in the phototransistor array the situation is a little different where the power dissipation of an active-pixel-sensor APS array is partially relying on the desired readout rate. Therefore, the common pixel-biasing load on each column and the analog line drivers primarily determines the power coupled with the readout. The measured power consumption can be defined by taking the average analog power dissipation from the pixel source-follower and the line driver based on the following formula [20]:

$$P_{diss} = 2F_rMV_{dd}(C_{col}\Delta V_{col} + 2\alpha C_{load}\Delta V_{out}) \qquad (3.11)$$

Where "F_r" is the frame-rate, C_{col} is the capacitance at the bottom of the column, and M is the total number of pixels readouts. V_{dd} is the power supply voltage, ΔV_{col} is the maximum voltage change at the bottom of the column, ΔV_{out} is the maximum voltage change at the output of the circuit, C_{load} is the capacitance of the line driver and α is a parameter that indicates the number of operations per pixel that lies within a range of 2-4.

The total power dissipated in the pixel source followers and the analog line drivers can be determined by setting the following parameters: $\alpha = 4$, $F_r = 1000$ Hz, $M = 1024$, $C_{col} = 2$ pF, $C_{load} = 35$ pF, $V_{dd} = 3.3$ V, $\Delta V_{out} = 0.15$ V, and $\Delta V_{col} = 1$ V. The total power dissipation is about 300 µW. The average power consumed in the pixel source followers is approximately 13.5 µW, and the power consumed in the subsequent line drivers is around 284 µW. The power dissipated in the digital timing and control circuits is highly considered through the design, therefore; it has become a figure of merit through the designer preparation. Table 3.3 shows different sensors with different specifications with respect to the recent work. By definition, the design's robustness can be determined as the ratio between the transistor length and the minimal length of the technology. Therefore, using CMOSP35 technology for resizing features of the design can also preserve the design's robustness, the smallest dimensions the better the robustness (i.e. from 0.35 micron, 0.5 micron, 0.8 micron, and 1.2 micron). Moreover, decreasing the area by using CMOSP35 technology declines the cost. Power consumption that depends on the applied voltages and the area of the features in the design also decreases. Therefore, the most updated technology utilized leads to improve the three main performance criteria: area, power consumption, and speed.

Table 3.3   Power consumption with respect to other technologies

CMOS Technology	Power supply	Phototransistor Array/ (pixel)	Pixel area/(μm^2)	Power Consumption	Reference No.
CMOSP35	3.3 V	32 by 32	40.1x 41.7	300 μW	Book
SOS 0.5	3.3 V	32 by 32	40 x 40	250 μW	[18]
MOSIS1.2	5.0 V	256 x 256	NA	3-5 mW	[20]
AMIS1.5	5 V	20 x 26	54 x 58	5.6 mW	[21]
AMS 0.8	3.0 V	12 x 63	50 x 350	60 mW	[22]
CMOS 0.8	5.0 V	256 x 256	NA	52-400 mW	[23]
CMOS 1.2	5 V	64 x 64	24 x 24	736 μW	[24]

3.5   Layout of one phototransistor pixel

The phototransistor of 32 by 32 arrays was integrated in the chip die that measures 1210.8 μm by 1318.4 μm. Note that the dimension of each pixel measures 40.2 μm by 41.775 μm. Figure 3-14 shows the layout of the phototransistor pixel. Figure 3-15a shows the layout of a phototransistor pixel along with the corresponding cross section. The vertical phototransistor is the utmost responsivity of the photodetectors available in the standard CMOS process that is provided by CMC where it is formed by the p-active (emitter)/n-well (base)/p-substrate (collector).

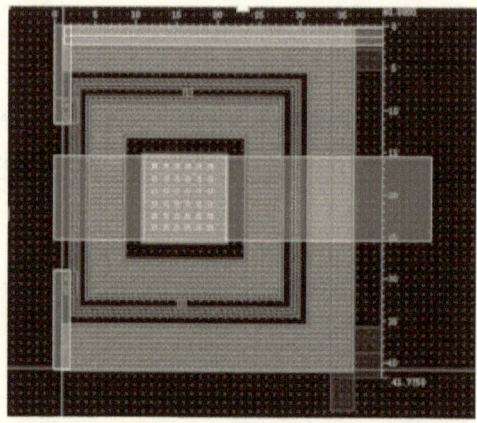

Figure 3-14 Layout of one phototransistor pixel.

Figure 3-15b shows the polysilicon grid that covers the n-well (base) forming a ring around the p-substrate (collector) contact.

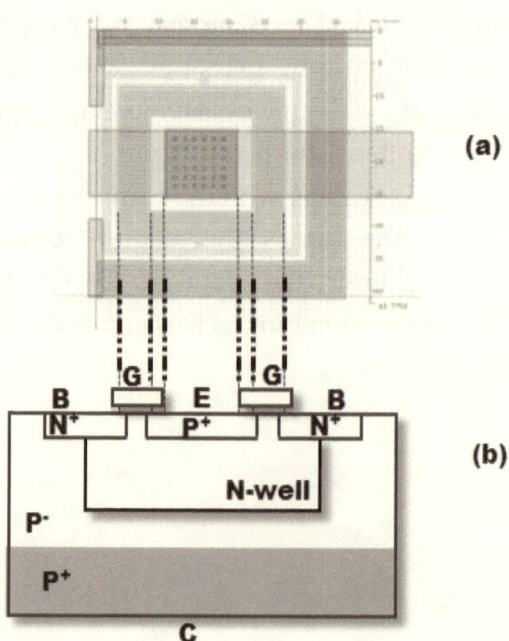

Figure 3-15 Layout view and corresponding cross-section of VPNP:
a) Layout view, b) Corresponding cross-section.

To avoid any formation of parasitic P+/N+ junctions in the thin polysilicon gate layer, gate contacts were added over the polysilicon ring; Figure 3-15a. The importance of the polysilicon grid that acts as a fourth terminal to PNP device is to increase the depletion region by setting it to the maximum potential, which leads to allowing the excess generated photo-carriers easily to flow to the p-active region (emitter). One of the best advantages of the phototransistor over the photodiode is that the photocurrent, which is generated through its operation, is adequately high.

3.6 The detector block operation

A high-sensitive biosensor based on VPNP phototransistors converts the optical signals into electrical current signals and at the end readouts the signal as a DC voltage signal. In essence, the biosensor is composed of four stages as shown in Figure 3-16. There is a phototransistor array stage where the optical signal converts to an electrical current signal. Then there is a current to voltage converter stage where the signal converts to a voltage signal. There is also an amplification stage where the voltage signal is amplified.

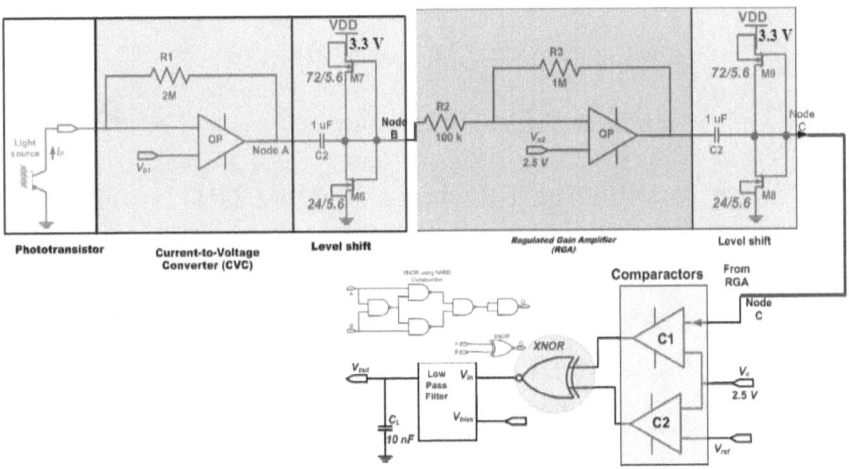

Figure 3-16 The optical biosensors stages.

At the last stage, a nonlinear phase detector provides a DC voltage signal proportional to the phase shift between the detected optical signal and a fixed reference sinusoidal signal that is obtained from a standard function generator. This optical sensor uses a new nonlinear phase detector that was proposed by Leo Yao *et. al* [25][26]. The proposed phase detector stage as shown in Figure 3-17 is composed of two comparators each implemented by standard wide-swing differential amplifiers. These are plugged into XNOR input gate, which is implemented by a standard digital gate [32] that ties its output to the input of a tunable low-pass filter stage, which transforms the phase difference into a DC voltage (V_{out}).

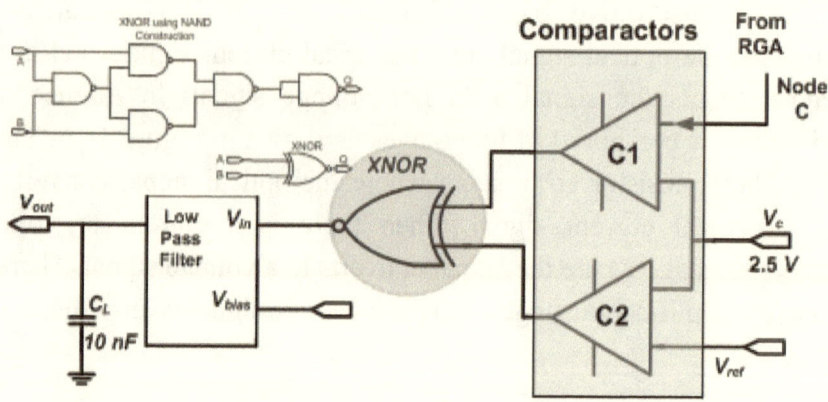

Figure 3-17 A nonlinear phase shift topology.

The low pass filter stage as shown in Figure 3-18, is built up as a voltage follower with V_{bias} as a controlling voltage. Through the duty cycle (D) of V_{in} at the high pulse period there is a source current charging the load capacitor; C_L and at the low-pulse period there is a sink current discharging. C_L is considered to be in nano range; (C_L = 10 nF), with the intention that the voltage alteration in C_L can be disregarded during the duty cycle.

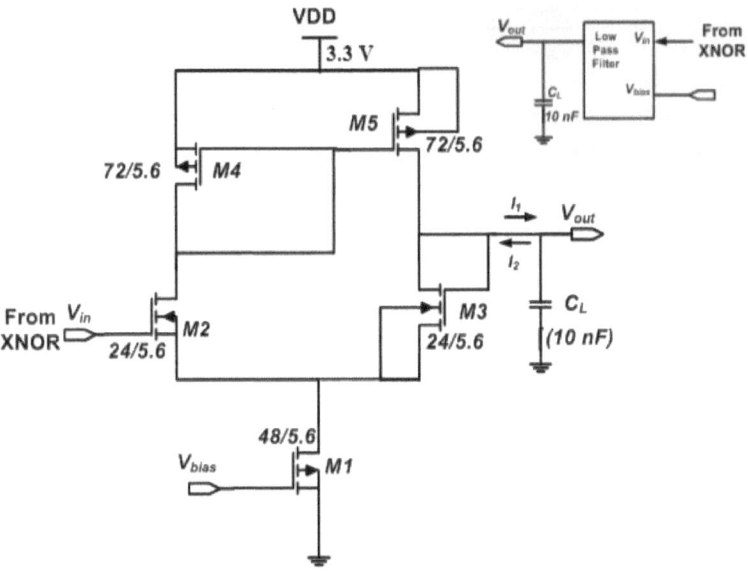

Figure 3-18 Schematic of low-pass-filter circuit in the phase detector structure.

3.7 Transduction and amplification

The mechanism of these stages rely on the pulse period of the input voltage that is charging/discharging the load capacitor; C_L. When the pulse is on the high level then a source current I_1 charges the load capacitor. However, when the pulse is on the low level a sink current I_2 discharges the load capacitor C_L. The generated photocurrent is usually weak and unreadable, for that reason, special care in setting the requirements for the design is essential. Transduction and amplification of the signal is a process, which takes place in between the input and output of the transducer. This process has been performed using the current-to-voltage converter (CVC); Figure 3-19 and the regulated gain amplifier (RGA); Figure 3-20 to amplify the signal and make it readable with good accuracy along with two voltage level shifters as shown in Figure 3-16.

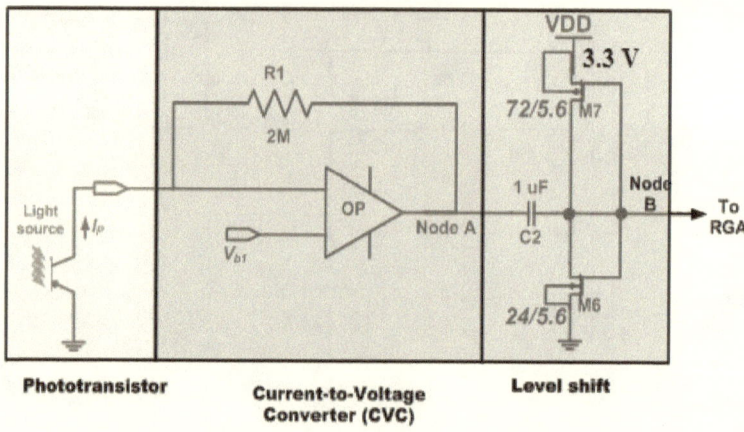

Figure 3-19 The current-voltage convertor stage.

The type of the TIA chosen in this work is a high-gain rail-to-rail folded-cascade op-amp as shown in Figure 3-2 with built-in feedback resistor, R_1 = 2M ohm. While the input signals of the CVC stage is connected to TIA amplifier is the photocurrent (I_p). This current is produced by the phototransistor array. The output signal from this stage is composed of two components; AC and DC components. The DC component is usually not that important and it is not taken into account; it is a byproduct of the biasing circuit. The AC component is the signal that is considered and recorded because of the phase information of the sinusoidal modulated luminescence signals. Afterward, the AC component as an output of the CVC stage feeds to the next stage to be amplified using the regulated gain amplifier (RGA) as shown in Figure 3-16. The characteristics of the RGA are similar to the high-gain rail-to-rail folded-cascade operational amplifier that the CVC is made of. The function of the RGA lies on regulating the gain up to double the input supply voltage through two built-in resistors; R_2 =100 kΩ and R3 =1 MΩ. The output frequency heavily depends on the concentration of pathogen cells. The higher the concentration of pathogens, the higher the intensity of the light output generated by the sensing surface, the higher the generated photodetector current. From the electrical point of view, the higher photodetector current that is produced means that there is a lower integration period, which means that there is an increase of the output frequency.

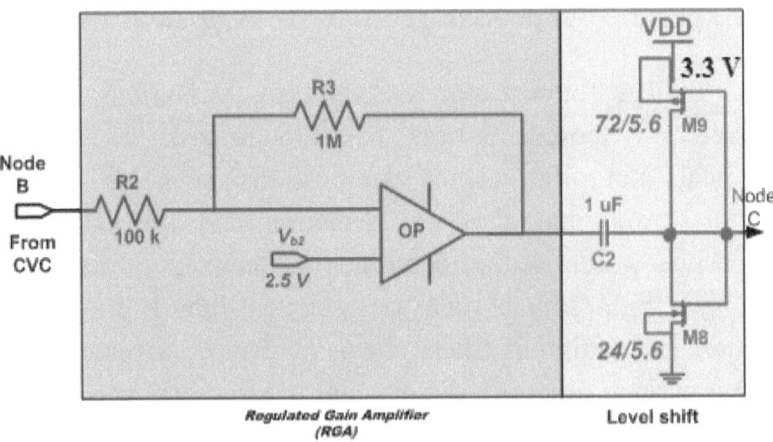

Figure 3-20 Regulated gain amplifier (RGA) stage.

The opposite of this process happens for the lower concentration of pathogens, which defines the performance of the transducer through showing the capability to sense very low concentration of bacterial pathogens cells. The minimum detectable signal (MDS) for the transducer is considered as a significant specification that can be defined by Eq.(3.12):

$$MDS \propto \frac{1}{\sqrt{t_{int}}} \qquad (3.12)$$

The phototransistor and the signal-processing circuit play a crucial role in this process. As a result, the longer the integration time, the more the weaker signal can be detected. When there is a long integration time, the comparator should be set for the specific voltage that should be applied to allow it to act in accordance with the input common-mode range of the comparator that should be experimentally specified. When designing the biosensing system, the lower the noise of the system the higher the performance of the transducer. This system would be capable of avoiding the influence of the noise on MDS that generates from the signal-processing unit [27].

3.8 Experimental procedures and MLoC system Validation

The optical fluorescence spectroscopy technology is widely employed for biosensors and has modernized the biological, biomedical and life science applications such as genomics, proteomics, and single-molecule detection [28]. Basically; optical fluorescence spectroscopy combines a number of components including a light source such as lasers or light emitting diodes, excitation and emission filters, focusing lenses, a pinhole, and a pumping syringe, microfluidic channel, microtubes, and an optical table as shown in Figure 3-21. The main function of the filters is to obscure the excitation light but they are translucent to the emission wavelength, therefore they are selected to go with the absorption and emission profiles of the required fluorescent dye. The consequential fluorescence from the illuminated light is detached from the illumination light thus the residual light is measured at the detector [29].

3.8.1 Experimental setup

The fluorescence spectroscopy schematic diagram setup of the assembled microfluidic glass/polymer substrate is integrated with the CMOS phototransistor biosensor as shown in Figure 3-21. The entire system afterwards is wrapped in polymethyl-methacrylate (PMMA) for packaging that aims to protect the device from the top and bottom from any external influences, which may fracture and damage the transducer. The microfluidic chip attaches to the biosensor through microfluidic tubing using fluidic inlet and outlet ports on the microfluidic channel where the electrical connection to the biosensor is provided by wiring the electrical pads of the optical chip to the PCB board.

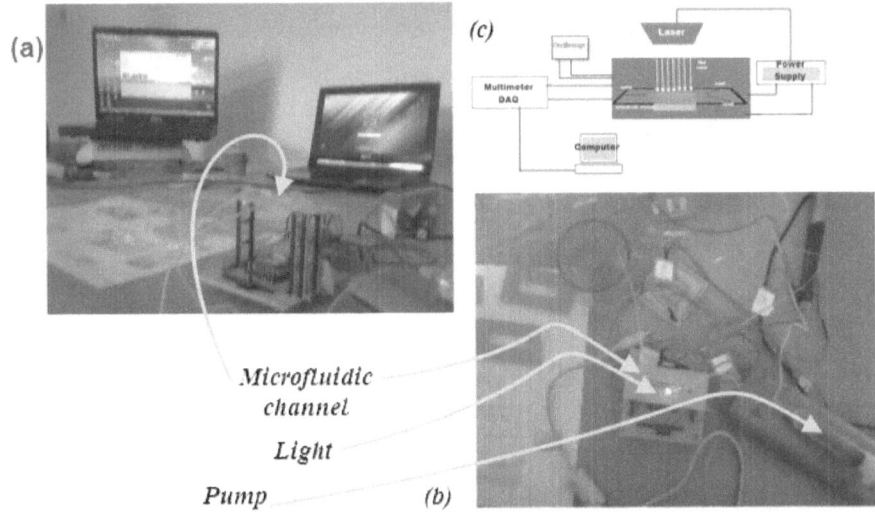

Figure 3-21 Optical setup and MLoC system validation.

A software user interface is developed using Labview to access the CMOS sensors' signals through the Data Acquisition (DAQ) multimeter card (National Instruments, 6024E) that feeds the PC for further signal analysis. A syringe pump is used to introduce and control particle samples into the channels of the microfluidic chip. Flow control in the microchannel is achieved by means of a high precision syringe pump in blowing mode connected to the channel inlet. Blowing mode allows introducing the particle suspension by simple pipetting into the outlet reservoir of the microfluidic chip holder. The system starts recording the data in real-time scanning once the corresponding section in the microfluidic channel is homogeneously filled. In time, the flow keeps running and the system keeps recording the data that refers to the concentration of the media [30].

3.8.2   CMOS microchip instrument

The phototransistor chip in this work was fabricated using the CMOSP35 process available through the CMC system. The entire chip die area is 2.23 mm x 3.04 mm and the phototransistor core area is only 1210.8 µm by 1318.4 µm, while each phototransistor pixel is 40.20 µm by 41.775 µm. The layout of the entire phototransistor system is shown in Figure 3-22 where the CMOS microchip is a single integrated circuit (IC) package that contains a phototransistor 32 by 32 arrays. The optical transducer consists of a vertical phototransistor array (VPTA), a current-to-voltage converter, an amplifier, a band-pass filter and a phase detector. The vertical phototransistor is formed by the p-active (emitter)/n-well (base)/p-substrate (collector), and has one of the utmost responsivity of the photodetectors available in standard CMOS process. The advantages of the CMOS-based system include its operation using low supply voltages and low cost of fabrication.

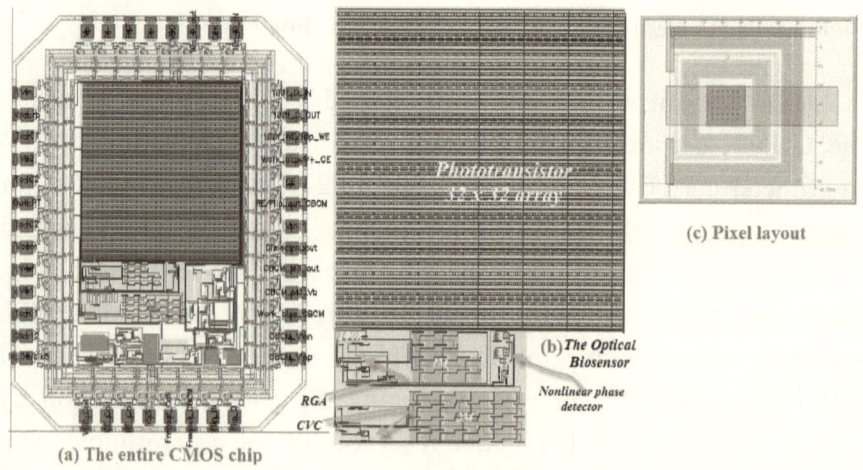

(c) Pixel layout

(b) The Optical Biosensor

Nonlinear phase detector

RGA

CVC

(a) The entire CMOS chip

Figure 3-22 The layout of the CMOS IC for photosensing device.

A National Instruments DAQ516 PCMCIA card is installed in a laptop computer provided with digital I/O lines and an analog-to-digital conversion channel so that the CMOS microchip detection elements were individually accessed and read out. A custom written software interface constructed with the Labview software controlled the data acquisition process for the CMOS microchip system.

3.8.3 Phage immobilization and protocol

The biomolecular recognition has to have immobilization antibodies on a good substrate such as gold along with a highly ordered molecular layer to have consistent capacitance measurements. The functionalities of biochips were used to detect different cancer markers. There are immobilization procedures that involve physical adsorption, covalent immobilization, and entrapment. Each protocol has an assortment of advantages and inconveniences depend on the nature of the functionalized surfaces of the sensing techniques that will apply to it. To get the receptor-ligand binding to match and work successfully, the immobilization of the membrane-associated receptors and the immobilization onto a sensor surface should be selected specifically and precisely to make certain that the receptor remains vigorous. For that reason some common protocols can be followed to accomplish this procedure certainly [31]:

1. Clean the chips three times with ethanol and dry with air.
2. Immerse the chips in 1mM Mercaptoundecanoic acid in ethanol for 24 hours for 20 ml of ethanol we need 0.0044g of Mercaptoundecanoic acid:
3. $\frac{1\ mml}{1000\ ml} \times \frac{1\ mol}{1000\ mml} \times \frac{218.36\ g}{1\ mol} \times 20\ ml = 0.0044\ g$
4. Wash the chips five times with ethanol and then dry with air.
5. Immerse the chip with EDC/NHS 1.15 g EDC in 15 ml high purity water, 200 mg NHS in 15 ml high quality water. Prepare EDC/NHS as required only as it decomposes very quickly. Required: For 10 ml of DI water, 0.77 g required of EDC, and 133.33 mg of NHS. Then the chip immersed for 1 hour.
6. Wash the chips five times with water and then three times with phosphate buffer.
7. Incubate the recognition elements with the activated surface for three hours with shaking. Wash 5-7 times with phosphate buffer.

8. Then block the surface with 1 mg/ml (Bovine Serum Albumin) BSA in phosphate buffer. BSA is used to block the surface to improve non-specific adsorption of the bacteria to the 1-hexadecanethiol.

9. The control surface will be exactly the same procedure as above except replace the BSA instead of recognition elements in step (6).

3.8.4 Bacteria preparation protocol

E. coli 12 and wild-type T4 bacteriophages were prepared at Biophage Pharma Inc. (Montreal, Canada).

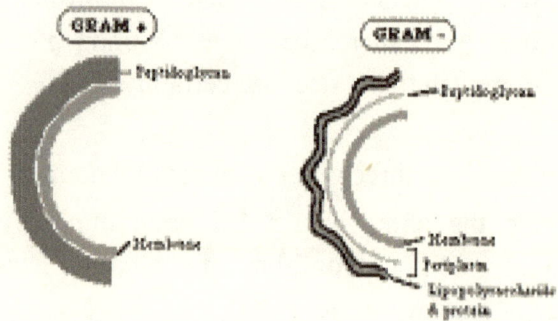

Figure 3-23 The structure of Gram-positive bacteria, and Gram-negative bacteria.

Escherichia coli are a Gram-negative bacterium that is commonly found in the lower intestine of warm-blooded organisms (endotherms). Most E. coli strains are harmless, but some, such as serotype O157:H7, can cause serious food poisoning in humans, and are occasionally responsible for costly product recalls [32]. The gram reaction relies on the structure of the bacterial cell wall, and it is sited in two categories as shown in Figure 3-23. In Gram-positive bacteria, the layer of peptidoglycan, which forms the outer layer of the cell, traps the purple crystal violet stain. In Gram-negative bacteria, the outer membrane prevents the stain from reaching the peptidoglycan layer in the periplasm. The outer membrane is then permeabilized by acetone treatment, and the pink safranin counter stain is trapped by the peptidoglycan layer [33].

3.8.5   Design and Fabrication (MFC)

The sensing layer represented by the microfluidic channel (MFC) is a foremost element in the optical spectroscopy detection process. The MFC can be either fluorescence-based or Label-free techniques. Fluorescence-based detection has more sensitivity than label-free techniques [34]. Therefore, this technique is suitable for biological application and particularly for tumor markers due to tiny sample volume and high sensitivity required. Microfluidic channel was designed and fabricated using soft photolithography technique in different styles; coated fully or partially by gold:

i.   Double glass slices adhered to each other leave a significant gap in between, making a channel. The channel is provided with two inlets and outlet, as shown in Figure 3-24

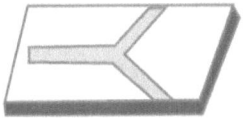

Figure 3-24 Microfluidic channel.

ii.   Microfluidic channels were fabricated using PDMS with one inlet and one outlet, and others were fabricated with two inlets and one outlet. The outcome was suitable results.

iii.   Microfluidic channels were fabricated by etching glass using a mixture of phosphoric acid (H_3PO_4), (or HF can be another option), then coated by gold. The outcome of this technique was unclear because of the roughness on the surface.

iv.   Microfluidic channels are fabricated by etching Si using TMAH, and then coated by gold. The results were clear. [35].

Soft photolithography technique is used for designing and fabricating a Microfluidic channel as shown in Figure 3-25; that is coated fully or partially by gold. Figure 3-26 illustrates MFC with three inlets and one outlet.

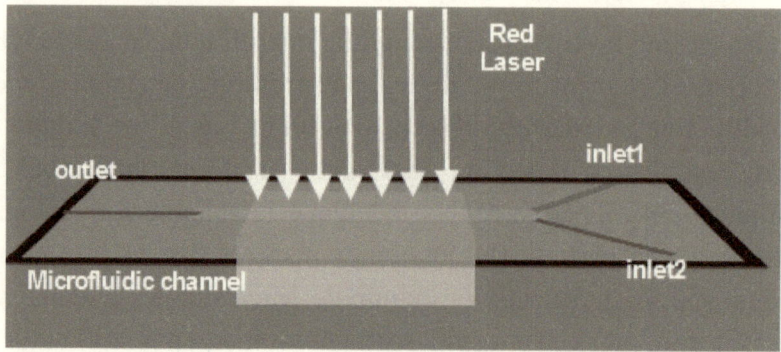

Figure 3-25 MFC after shining the system with red laser.

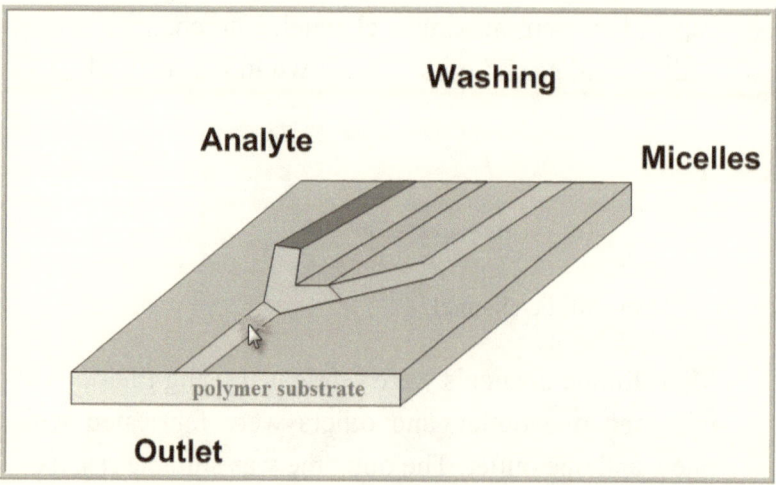

Figure 3-26 Microfluidic channel with three inlets and outlet.

MFC cleaning is an essential step, therefore, the sensing layer should be cleaned in either a piranha solution (mixture of 3:1 of H_2SO_4 and H_2O_2) or using an electrochemical process. The second technique is more reliable but the first is less expensive, more rapid and available and easy to prepare in the laboratory.

3.9 Optical biosensor on MLoC System Validation

3.9.1 Bacterial pathogens results

E. coli 12 was used to act as a target for a detection process in different concentration and types. Figure 3-21 demonstrates a schematic view of the experimental setup. It involves the integrated CMOS microchip system, an external laser source; 473 nm blue laser; (0.6-25mW Aquarius Series Blue Laser), and a pinhole was used to eliminate extraneous light from the laser. The laser beam was focused onto the optical chip array using a capillary holder that is adjusted using a translational stage so that the laser beam is passed through the center of the microfluidic channel (MFC). Fluorescence from the MFC was detected with the CMOS microchip that was laid on it. Thereafter, the data was collected using a 2700-Multimeter/Data Acquisition System and National Instruments DAQ516 PCMCIA card installed in a laptop computer. A band pass optical filter (cut-off position: 510 nm, Edmund Industrial Optics) was attached on the CMOS microchip to eliminate the laser scattering.

3.9.1.1 Before encapsulation the chip

Figure 3-27 shows the fluorescence detection of E-coli obtained with the CMOS microchip system after the MFC is filled with high concentration of bacteria 10^9 using microfluidic pumps. The laser beam irradiation onto MFC was well controlled.

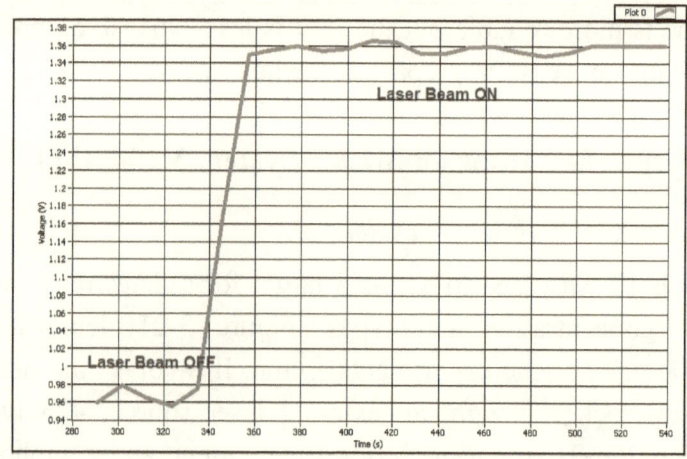

Figure 3-27 Optical response of phototransistors array in the CMOS microchip OFF/ON state.

When the laser beam was irradiating MFC, the phototransistors showed obvious optical response. The dark current signal was obtained when there was no laser beam irradiation onto MFC. The fluorescence intensities of E-coli 12 decreased while DI water was pumping through MFC. The bacteria detection was performed after this optical adjustment for the detection of the highest fluorescence signal.

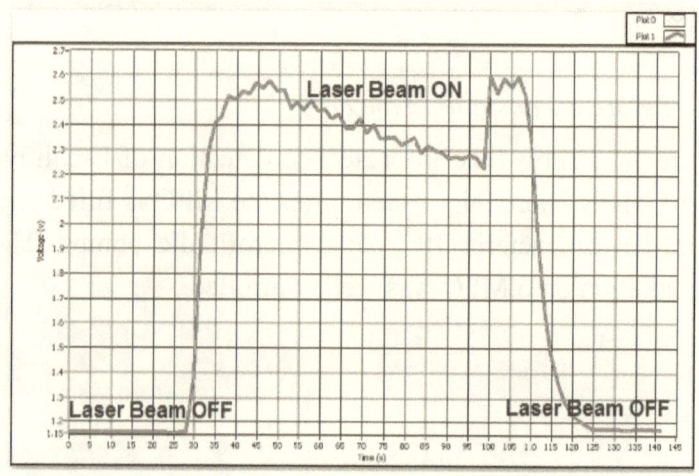

Figure 3-28 The entire detection cycle.

A full cycle was recorded, as shown in Figure 3-28, starting with the dark current signal; when the laser beam is off. This is followed by high concentration of bacteria where the laser is ON then pumping DI water through this step. The signal that resulted was a little bit higher than the previous one because of residual bacteria. High concentration of bacteria is then pumped through this step, after which we switch the laser beam OFF.

After the IC microchip system showed the remarkable results, we applied fluorescent Material to check on the response behavior and performance of phototransistors arrays. Figure 3-29 shows the profiles because of DI water and fluorescent Material, where the reproducibility of the experiment was observed.

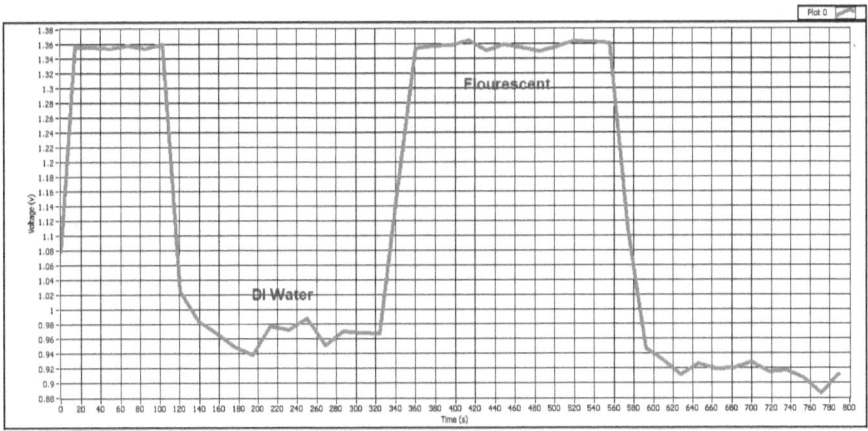

Figure 3-29 The phototransistors were used to record the fluorescence signals of DI water and fluorescence material as a reference.

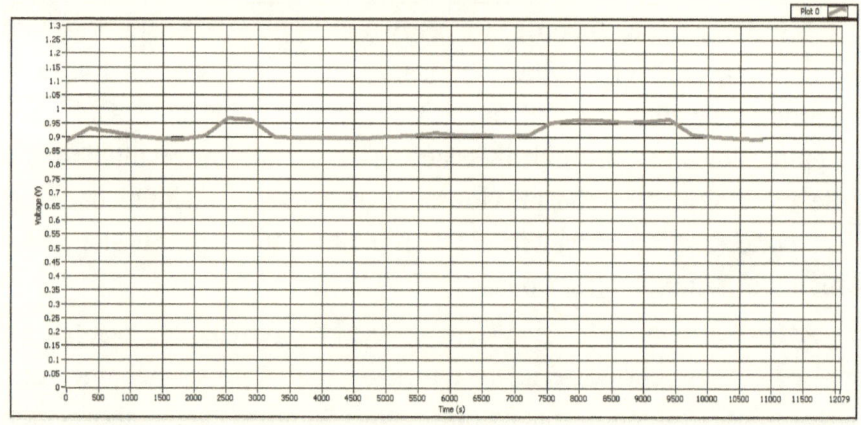

Figure 3-30 The fluorescence signal recorded for the positive bacteria, with high concentration and DI water, respectively.

The bacteria E-coli 12 were prepared in two categories; Gram-positive and Gram-negative. A significant detection voltage was observed when the mixture (bacteria and LB) was pumped through the MFC and the microchip's response was recorded. Figure 3-30 shows the profile because of the flowing DI water through MFC, then the bacteria in LB media pumping with high concentration (10^9). Gram-positive type of bacteria is used in this case; a voltage around 95 mV is detected.

3.9.1.2 *After encapsulation the chip*

The experiment was repeated after the optical chip was encapsulated using Norland Optical Adhesives. NOA60 are clear, colorless, one part adhesives that contain no solvents. When exposed to ultraviolet light, they gel in seconds and full cure in minutes to give a tough, resilient bond.

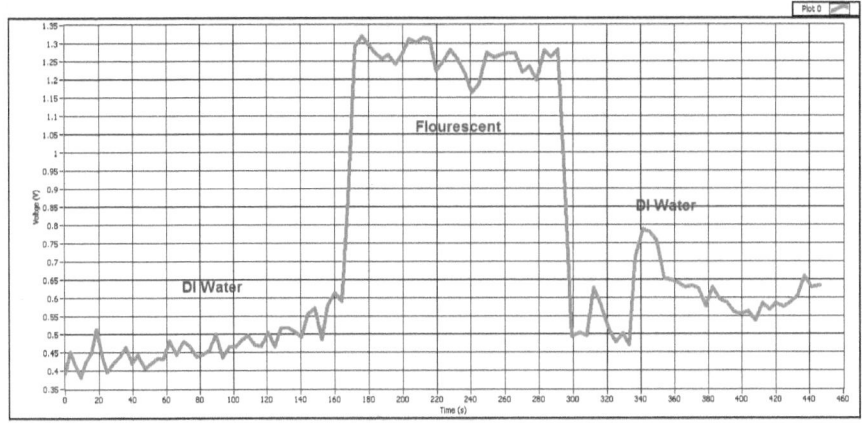

Figure 3-31 The phototransistors were used to record the fluorescence signals of DI water and fluorescence material after encapsulating the microchip.

These adhesives are designed for fast, precision bonding where low strain and optical clarity are required; the following experiments have been done. The experiment was repeated but after the microchip has modified by encapsulating it using NOA60. A profile was recorded as a result of the flowing DI water through MFC and then the fluorescent material respectively. Figure 3-31 shows this result without recording any significant difference from the previous experiment.

Figure 3-32 shows a profile because of the flowing DI water and bacteria with high concentration (positive type) respectively. A voltage was detected around 150 mV. The bacteria is in two different categories; Gram-positive and Gram-negative. This was also considered in this work and a profile as shown in Figure 3-23 demonstrated the different structure of each category,

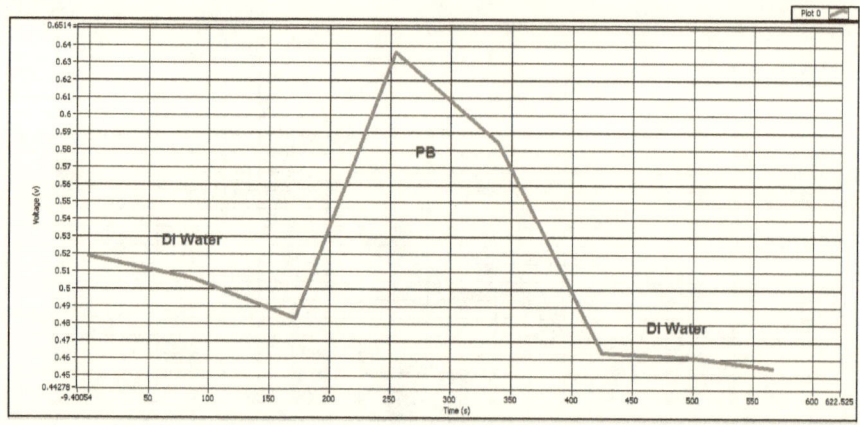

Figure 3-32 The fluorescence signal recorded for the positive bacteria, with high concentration and DI water, respectively, after encapsulation.

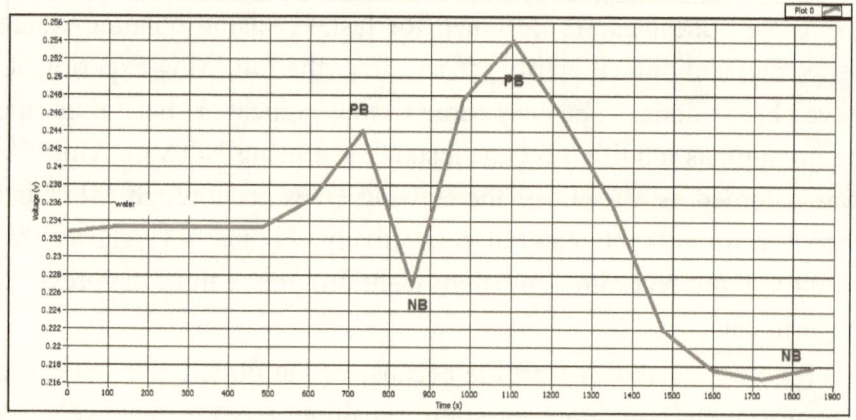

Figure 3-33 The fluorescence signal for negative and positive bacteria.

Figure 3-33 is a remarkable observation because of the DI water and the pumping bacteria; positive type (BP) then the pumping Bacteria; negative type; (BN) with high concentration respectively.

3.9.2 Summary

Optical-based technique is specifically designed, fabricated, and experimentally validated for realizing a new generation of multi-labs on a single chip (MLoC) system. Attributable to its compact design and multiplex capability, the integrated optical sensor as a part of the MLoC chip worked successfully and provided high-gain and throughput analysis as a tool for the detection of bacteria in medical diagnosis and bacterial pathogen based on its compactness, low cost, multiplex capability, selectivity and sensitive method. The integrated MLoC system as a detector expects to be compatible with conventional microfabricated devices to allow more rapid and high throughput analysis. In the light of the definition of originality aforementioned in "*section* 1.4", the optical techniques fill in the first category where the ideas have been previously published. The design in the literature made of exposed area 16 × 16 arrays, the technology that used was AMIS 1.5 μm, and power supply 5 V but the tools for MLoC system are definitely different. In this design, the technology that used is CMOSP35, the exposed area is 32 × 32 arrays, and power supply is 3.3 V. As it is well known that, the exposed area of the biosensor is matter and the wider exposed area improves significantly its sensitivity. Furthermore, the lower power supply to the less power consumption produced and this situation applies on all of the biosensor in the MLoC system, as the power supply is 3.3 V.

3.10 References

[1]   Simpson, Michael L.; Sayler, Gary S.; Nivens, David; Ripp, Steve; Paulus, Michael J.; Jellison, Gerald E., "Bioluminescent bioreporter integrated circuits (BBICs) Whole-Cell Environmental Monitoring Devices" National Research Council, "Existing and Potential Standoff Explosives Detection Techniques". The National Academies Press, 2004.

[2] Sara Wallin & Anna Pettersson & Henric Östmark, Alison Hobro, "Laser-based standoff detection of explosives: a critical review", Anal Bioanal Chem, 395:259-274, 2009.

[3] Steven Ripp, Scott Moser, Brandon Weathers, Sam Caylor, Benjamin Blalock, Syed Islam, and Gary Sayler, "Bioluminescent bioreporter integrated circuit (BBIC) sensors", Bio Micro and Nanosystems Conference,. BMN '0615-18 Jan. 2006 Page(s):59-60, 2006.

[4] Gary S Sayler, Michael L Simpson, Chris D Cox, "Emerging foundations: nano-engineering and bio-microelectronics for environmental biotechnology Current Opinion in Microbiology", Volume 7, Issue 3, Pages 267-273, June 2004.

[5] Steven Ripp, Gary S. Sayler, "Advanced Bioreporter Technologies For Targeted Sensing Of Chemical And Biological Agents",

[6] Ibtisam E. Tothill, "Biosensors for cancer markers diagnosis" Seminars in Cell & Developmental Biology, *Volume* **20**, Issue 1, Pages 55-62, February 2009.

[7] Drezek R, Sokolov K, Utzinger U, Boiko I, Malpica A, Follen M, Richards-Kortum R, "Understanding the contributions of NADH and collagen to cervical tissue fluorescence spectra: modeling, measurements, and implications", J. Biomed Opt 2001, 6:385-396, 2001.

[8] Avraham Rasooly, "Moving biosensors to point-of-care cancer diagnostics", Biosensors and Bioelectronics, Volume 21, Issue 10, Pages 1847-1850, 15 April 2006.

[9] D. C. Latham, Lindholm, Hamilton, "Low-Frequency Operation of Four-Terminal Field-Effect Transistors", IEEE February 6, 1964.

[10] Søren J Sørensen, Mette Burmølle, Lars H Hansen, "Making bio-sense of toxicity: new developments in whole-cell biosensors", Current Opinion in Biotechnology, Volume 17, Issue 1, Pages 11-16, February 2006.

[11]   Robert C. Genn, "Practical Solid State Circuits", Jr., Prentice-Hall, ISBN 0-13-450643-X, 1983.

[12]   Adrio Communications Ltd, Ian Poole "Phototransistor", www.radio-electronics.

[13]   Matsumoto, Y. Hara, T. Kimura, Y., "CMOS photo-transistor array detection system for visual light identification (ID)", Networked Sensing Systems, INSS 2008, 5th International Conference on, page(s): 99 - 102 17-19 June 2008.

[14]   Voegeli, B.; Gray, P.; Dahlstrom, M.; Feilchenfeld, N.; Rainey, B.; Previti-Kelly, R.; St Onge, S.; Joseph, A.; Dunn, J.; "High Performance, Low Complexity Vertical PNP BJT Optimization for a 0.24 μm SiGe BiCMOS Technology", Silicon Monolithic Integrated Circuits in RF Systems, 2007, Page(s): 80-82.

[15]   E. Culurciello, "Three-dimensional phototransistors in 3D silicon-on-insulator technology", Electronics Letters, IEEE, Volume 43, Issue 7, Page(s):418-420, March 29 2007.

[16]   EG&G Optpelectronics, "Characteristics of Phototransistors", 1997.

[17]   V. A. Labusov, D. O. Selyunin, I. A. Zarubin and R. G. Gallyamov, "Measuring the quantum efficiency of multielement photodetectors in the spectral range between 180 and 800 nm", Optoelectronics, Instrumentation and Data Processing, Volume 44, Number 1 / February, 2008.

[18]   Joon Hyuk Park, Eugenio Culurciello, "Phototransistor Image Sensor in Silicon on Sapphire", in IEEE International Symposium on Circuits and Systems, ISCAS '08. Seattle, USA: IEEE, Page(s): 1416-1419, May 2008

[19]   Yoshinori Matsumoto, Takaharu Hara and Yohsuke Kimura, "Integrated CMOS photo-transistor array for visual light identification (ID)", ISDRS 2007, Dec. 12-14, College Park, MD, USA, 2007.

[20]   Nixon, R.H.; Kemeny, S.E.; Staller, C.O.; Fossum, E.R.; "256×256 CMOS active pixel sensor camera-on-a-chip", Solid-State Circuits Conference, 1996. Digest of Technical Papers. 42nd ISSCC., 1996 IEEE International 1996, Page(s): 178 - 179, 440.

[21]   Lei Yao, Mohamad Hajj Hassan, Vamsy Chodavarapu, Arghavan Shabani, Beatrice Allain, Mohammed Zourob, Rosemonde Mandeville, "CMOS Imager Microsystem for Multi-Bacteria Detection", IEEE 2006.

[22]   P. Fischer, J. Hausmann, M. Overdick, B. Raith, N. Wermes, L. Blanquart, V. Bonzom, P. Delpierre, "A counting pixel readout chip for imaging applications", Nuclear Instruments and Methods in Physics Research Section A: Accelerators, Spectrometers, Detectors and Associated Equipment, Volume 405, Issue 1, Pages 53-59, 1 March 1998.

[23]   Decker, S.; McGrath, D.; Brehmer, K.; Sodini, C.G.; "A 256×256 CMOS imaging array with wide dynamic range pixels and column-parallel digital output", Solid-State Circuits, IEEE Journal of Volume: 33, Issue: 12, Page(s): 2081-2091, 1998.

[24]   Zhimin Zhou, Bedabrata Pain, Eric R. Fossum, "CMOS Active Pixel Sensor with On-Chip Successive Approximation Analog-To-Digital Converter", IEEE Transactions On Electron Devices, Vol. 44, No. 10, October 1997.

[25]   L. Yao, Abdullah. Tashtoush, E. Ghafer-Zadeh, R. Mandeville, V. Chodavarapu, "CMOS Imaging of Biological and Chemical Sensor Microarrays", Presented at the Canadian Institute for Photonics Innovation (CIPI) Annual Meeting, Quebec city, May 2009.

[26]   Lei Yao, Rifat Khan, Vamsy P. Chodavarapu, Vijay S. Tripathi, and Frank V. Bright, "Sensitivity-Enhanced CMOS Phase Luminometry System Using Xerogel-Based Sensors",

IEEE Transactions On Biomedical Circuits And Systems, PP. 1-8, 2009.

[27]   W. Sansen, D. De wachter, l. Callewaert, M. Lambrechts and a Claes, "A Smart Sensor for the Voltammetric Measurement of Oxygen or Glucose Concentrations", Sensors and Actuators, BI 298-302, 1990.

[28]   Michael Schäferling and Stefan Nagl, "Optical technologies for the read out and quality control of DNA and protein microarrays", Analytical and Bioanalytical Chemistry, Volume 385, Number 3 / June, 2006.

[29]   Kim Sapsford, Chris Rowe Taitt, Frances S. Ligler, "Planar waveguides for fluorescence biosensors", Optical Biosensors (Second Edition), 2008, Pages 139-184.

[30]   Noriyuki Nakamura, Tae-Kyu Lim, Jae-Mun Jeong, Tadashi Matsunaga, "Flow immunoassay for detection of human chorionic gonadotrophin using a cation exchange resin packed capillary column", Analytica Chimica Acta, Volume 439, Issue 1, 17 July 2001, Pages 125-130.

[31]   L. Gervais, M. Gela, B. Allain, M. Tolba, L. Brovko, M. Zourob, R. Mandeville, M. Griffiths, S. Evoy, "Immobilization of biotinylated bacteriophages on biosensor surfaces", Sensors and Actuators B 125, 615-621, 2007.

[32]   Vesela I. Chalova, Sujata A. Sirsat, Corliss A. O'Bryan, Philip G. Crandall and Steven C. Ricke, "Escherichia coli, an Intestinal Microorganism, as a Biosensor for Quantification of Amino Acid Bioavailability", Sensors 2009, 9, 7038-7057; 2009.

[33]   Magdalena Gabig-Ciminska, Marcin Los, Anders Holmgren, J€org Albers, Agata Czyz, Reiner Hintsche, Grzegorz Wegrzyn, and Sven-Olof Enfors, "Detection of bacterial pathogen DNA using an integrated complementary metal oxide semiconductor microchip system with capillary array electrophoresis", Analytical Biochemistry 324, 84-91, 2004.

[34]   Graciela M. Escandar, Patricia C. Damiani, Héctor C. Goicoechea, Alejandro C. Olivieri, "A review of multivariate calibration methods applied to biomedical analysis", Microchemical Journal, Volume 82, Issue 1, Pages 29-42, January 2006.

[35]   Tashtoush, A. Landsberger, LM; Essalik, A.; Kahrizi, M. Paranjape, M. Currie, JF; Pandy, A. "Experimental Characterization of the Si/Al/Tetramethylammonium Hydroxide System", Journal of the Electrochemical Society 148: (7) p. C456-C460, 2001

Chapter 4 - Electrochemical Impedance Spectroscopy for Electrochemical Sensing Biomolecules

4.1 Introduction

In medical biological and biotechnological applications, biochemical approaches and biological quantifications are of extreme importance. The changes in the surface that connects the sensing element to analyze the content of a biological sample at a tiny scale are the key requirements for the signal amplification and the general performance of electrochemical biosensors. The performance and sensitivity of the biosensor heavily depends on the surface type selection, the methodology of the electrochemical transducer, and the choice of the recognition receptor molecules. Electrochemical biosensors play an important role, therefore; it is considered a smart approach thanks to direct detection for a biological environment to an electronic signal. In biosensors, the optimization of the sensor response and the interpretation of its behavior are places of interest. The Electrochemical Biosensor is an analytical transducer that detects a biological response into a quantifiable and processed electrical signal. Typically, biosensors are built based on bioreceptors that specifically attach to the analyte. The bioreceptors have a surface architecture where a specific biological environment is present. On the other hand, the transducer component of the biosensor is where the signal is transformed to an electronic signal and amplified by an electronics circuit then processed to a physical parameter. The antibody works based on the sensing surface that determines the entire IDMA area. This becomes responsive to the presence of bacterial pathogens cells.

The EIS technique was introduced last century by Lorenz *et. al.* [1]. The measurement of this technique lies on applying a small *AC* voltage then measuring the response current. The complex impedance can be determined in case the applied voltage is over a range of frequency. Such results can be plotted using either Nyquist or bode diagrams depending on the analysis requirements. Electrochemical impedance spectroscopy is a powerful technique to develop biosensors that are capable to detect and analyze biomaterials' behavior. Moreover, these techniques are able to investigate and monitor the electrical properties, resulting from a specific process that occurs on the electrode/electrolyte interface due to biorecognition events. For instance, modifying the sensing surface by either protein immobilization or antibody-antigen (Ab-Ag) immunoreactions on the sensing surface leads to a change in the conductance of the electrodes. The double capacitance that is established between the sensing surface, represented by the IDMA, and the electrolyte can be measured using an EIS technique named as Faradaic impedance spectroscopy. Monitoring the immunoreactions occur in the space between the microelectrodes as well. [2]. The Electrochemical Impedance Spectroscopy (EIS) is an experimental method of characterizing electrochemical systems.

Biosensors are transducers that exploit biomolecular interactions to recognize biological media such as hormones, glucose, deoxyribonucleic acid and proteins. Biosensors in their simplest structure connect a biological recognition element, well known as the probe, with the sensing surface that performs transcription as a first step leading to the translation of the biorecognition event into a detectable then measured signal. The biological recognition element exploits the two main characteristics of biosensors; selectivity and specificity of the biological reactions either antibody-antigen (Ab-Ag) interactions in immunoassays or a molecular biology technique that measures the degree of genetic similarity between pools of DNA sequences [3]. Utilizing CMOS technology in the miniaturized electrochemical transducer makes this technique the utmost selectable method among the others for biological and biomedicine application due to its high performance and lower cost. Furthermore, electrochemical impedance spectroscopy (EIS) has the capability to endow free label detection, size, power consumption, real-time, simplicity and portable systems. The core of this technique lies on using a small device named potentiostat as shown in Figure 4-1 where the differential potential occurs in between the electrodes in simplicity; i.e. CE and RE translates to a measurable current at the work electrode. The measured value at the output is not confined by a current but it can take two forms. The first approach is called the Faradaic approach that uses a specific label. The second approach is called the non-Faradaic approach that is based on a label-free technique. The Faradaic approach is based on measuring the variation of the current flow across electrode-electrolyte interface in the light of Ohm's law. The non-Faradaic approach is based on measuring the variation of the current that results from the rise and fall of the charge on the sensing surface. The main drawback of the EIS technique is that it is almost confined in the DNA detection through the preparation step of the sensing surface named hybridization, where it was observed that some variation is established in between the active layer that is functionalized with probe molecules and the electrolyte [4].

The transducer is implemented using CMOSP35 technology, exploiting the advantages of the semiconductor fabrication processes by reducing the size of the device that can usually achieve a high-sensitivity electrochemical biosensor. Figure 4-2 illustrates the architecture of the electrochemical biosensors that is presented in this work and that builds on an active CMOS substrate. It mainly implies three units. The first unit is a voltage control unit representing the CMOS potentiostat. It is made of two operational amplifiers; one is a feedback amplifier for the reference electrode (RE) and it is connected to the other operational amplifiers through two nMOS transistors, where the output of the latter will connect to the CE terminal on the microfluidic cell (MFC). The second unit is the signal-processing unit. It is made of Current-to-Frequency converters (CFCs). This unit implies two operational amplifiers, one works as the integrator (TIA) and the other as a comparator connected through two nMOS transistors as switches. It also implies voltage reference V_{bias}, one-shot, and triggered flip-flop circuit. Finally, the off-chip active layer as a sensing surface, represents MCF made of interdigitated microelectrodes with three terminals; WE, CE and RE [5].

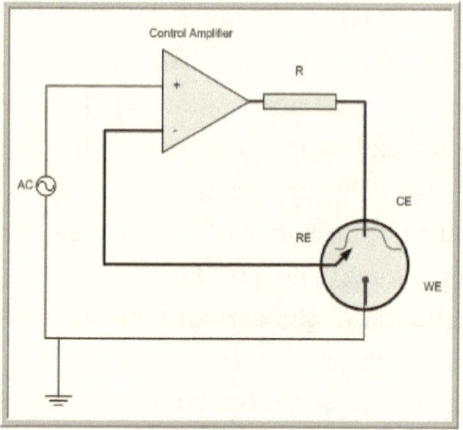

Figure 4-1   Basic Potentiostat scheme.

4.2   Electrochemical Biosensors - Sensor Principles and Architectures

Over the past decades, quite a lot of sensing models and related industrial devices have been in favor of biosensors applications. In medical, biological and biotechnological applications, biochemical approaches and biological quantifications are of extreme importance. On the other hand, the convolution of connecting an electronic device directly to a biological setting is very challenging because of altering the biological data straightforwardly to the processed electronic signal. Therefore, electrochemical biosensors play an important role in this domain as a smart approach thanks to direct detection for a biological environment to an electronic signal.

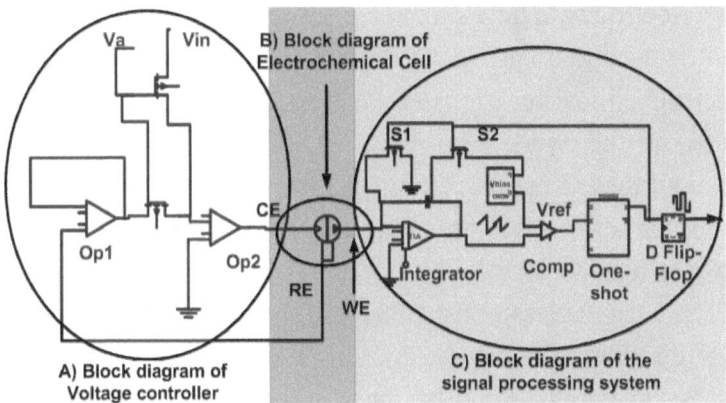

Figure 4-2   Electrochemical biosensor architecture.

4.3   Electrochemical Detection Techniques

Electrochemical immunosensors have the potential to make immunoassay easier and reduce the expense of clinic diagnosis. Besides, they are miniaturizable devices and they have computerizable detection due to their affinity ligand-based transducers that connect immunochemical responses to proper biosensors and have a handle on a state-of-the-art biomolecular breakdown. Electrochemical detection can be performed using the label reporter or it can be label-free. The detection process for biomolecular responses is the foremost sensitive due to the amplification given by the label through employing electroactive signal producing labels. This process requires the use of a label, such as fluorescent labeling, for sensing the biomolecular recognition between a ligand and its receptor, such as the antibody-antigen (Ab-Ag). The electrochemical technique can measure the generated electrical signals of the labeled species and carry out the output as impedance, capacitance or admittance [6].

4.4 CMOS-Integrated potentiostat behavior

Potentiostat is a feedback control system. Its operation requires a three-electrode configuration represented by working, reference and counter electrodes. The entire set is called the electrochemical cell. The cell is used to measure the flow of charges that are resulted from the electrochemical reactions at the electrode-electrolyte interface. In the case of the work electrode, where biomolecular probes are binding and the immunoreactions of interest take place are immersed alone in the electrolyte, no current flows through the electrode-electrolyte interface. Once the counter electrode (CE) is attached to the cell, a current is established accordingly. The current flow in the external circuit is due to the moving electrons between electrodes named as the Faradaic current and applied to Ohm's law where the movement of charges in the solution forms a double layer capacitance hence a displacement current is established and named as the non-Faradaic process. The situation is still ambiguous and it is not recognized at the surface of the two electrodes; work and counter. Therefore, a third electrode named the reference electrode (RE) is playing an important role by holding the electrode-electrolyte interface at a specific potential by adjusting externally applied potential V_{in}. The preferred potential between the working electrode and the counter electrode could then be defined accordingly. Finally, the electrochemical cell is under control and its behavior so far is clear and ready for measurements due to the potential in between the working electrode and the counter electrode that is attuned to set up a preferred cell potential V_{in} between the working electrode and the reference electrode. Afterwards, the reference electrode in the chip is tied to the high input impedance operational amplifier to ascertain that very low current flows through. The potentiostat test chip is fabricated using a TSMC standard CMOSP35 process provided by the CMC. The test chip is powered from nominal power-supply voltage of 3.3 V. Figure 4-2 shows the implementation of the potentiostat circuit that can be divided in three main parts. The first part to the left is the control voltage unit that represents the basic potentiostat function. The second part located on the right side is the signal-processing unit that has the integrator and comparator to translate the signal to frequency data then transmit the digital data off-chip. Therefore, the measurements can perform as frequency vs. time. The third part located in the middle is the microfluidic channel that implies interdigitated microelectrode arrays as a sensing surface. The overall size of the CMOS potentiostat chip sites is 500 μm by 380.6 μm. A CMOS-based EIS for chemical/biological sensing was introduced in many references [7][8]. However, in this work, significant effort has been made to improve the robustness and the performance of the individual components that the signal-processing circuitry comprises. In addition, the operation of the signal-processing system is modified to improve the overall quality. Figure 4-3 shows the block diagram of the implementation layout.

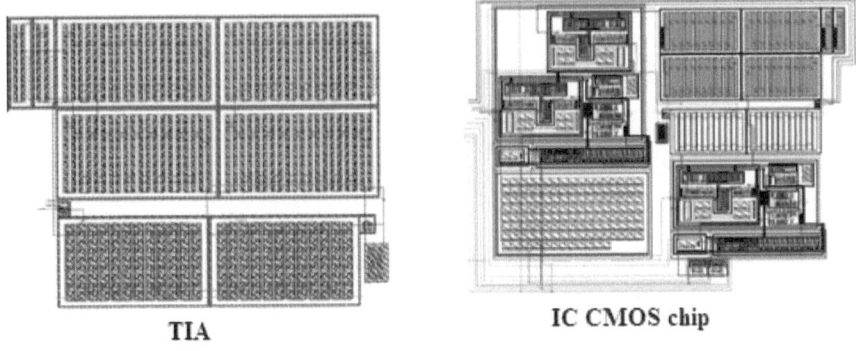

TIA

IC CMOS chip

Figure 4-3   The layout of the OP-Amp and the entire CMOS IC chip.

The CMOS IC chip consists of integrated CMOS potentiostat, the electrochemical cell and the signal-processing system. Figure 4-4 shows the architecture of the CMOS potentiostat. The signal-processing system shown in Figure 4-5, is the key component of the IC CMOS potentiostat.

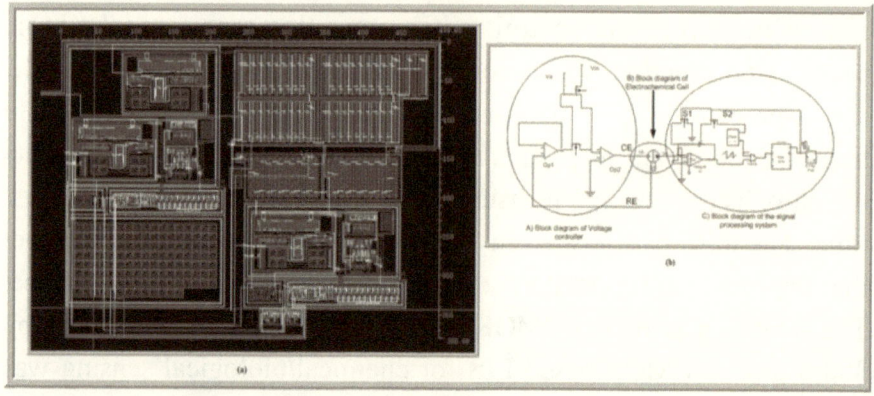

Figure 4-4   (a) Layout of IC CMOS chip (b) the architecture of the chip.

4.4.1   Signal-processing unit

The signal-processing unit is the key component of the impedance measurements system. The bioreporter sensing concentration of the bacterial pathogen presence in the microfluidic channel will modify the impedance of electrolyte (Z). In the light of Ohm's law:

$$I = \frac{V}{Z_T} \tag{4.1}$$

Where the total impedance Z_T is composed of two parts, the real part Z_{Re} and the imaginary part Z_{Im} described by the following equations:

$$Z_T = Z_{Re} + Z_{Im} \tag{4.2}$$

$$Z_{Re} = R \tag{4.3}$$

$$Z_{Im} = -\frac{1}{2\pi j f C} \tag{4.4}$$

Therefore, as the impedance decreases due to the high concentration, it increases the drawn current that flows through the working electrode. Such situation translates in to a lower integration period leading to increase the output frequency and vice versa in case of a lower concentration.

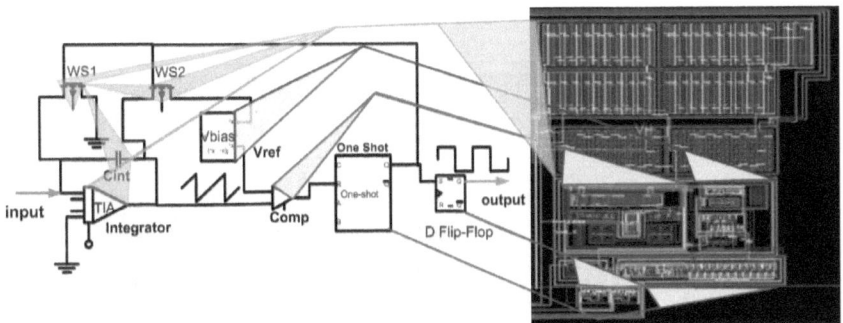

Figure 4-5   The signal-processing unit arctechtiture and layout.

The electrochemical-based impedance system is a useful sensing system for a very low concentration of an environmental biological domain. Consequently, the bioreceptor and the signal-processing circuit play an important role throughout the measurement process. The biosensor performance must have the capability to sense very low concentration of environmental pollutants where the minimum detectable signal (MDS) for the transducer is considered as a significant specification due to its capability to delineate the MDS that can be defined by [9]:

$$MDS \propto \frac{1}{\sqrt{t_{int}}} \tag{4.5}$$

Consequently, the longer the integration time, the weaker the signal detected. Potentiostat and the signal-processing circuit play a crucial role in this process. Therefore, to have a longer integration time, the comparator reference voltage should be set to a high enough value. The high voltage value imposes on the comparator to have a high input common-mode range. Note that the targeted voltage value is around 2.4 V. The biosensing system should be designed very carefully for low noise to avoid the influence of the noise on the MDS that generates from the signal-processing unit (SPU) and acts a CFC. [10]. Figure 4-6 shows the layout of the TIA and the whole IC CMOS potentiostat.

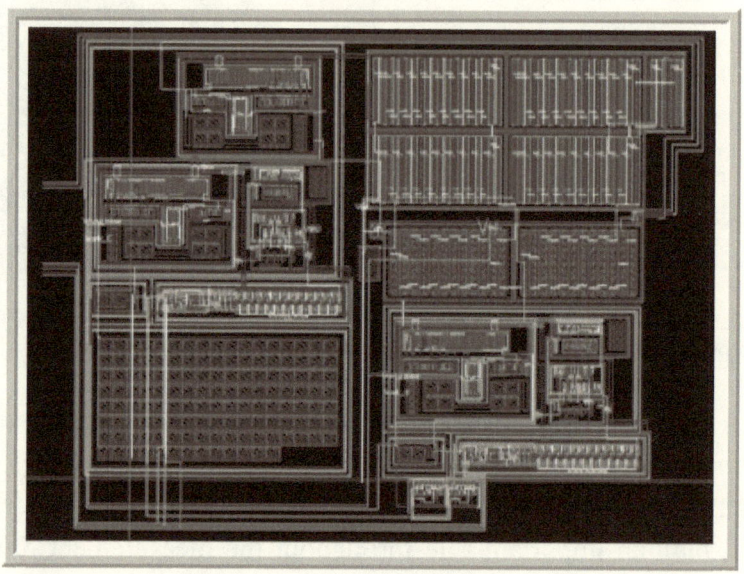

Figure 4-6   CMOS potentiostat layout.

By adding a specific resistor in series to the input of the integrator, the SPU converts the current from a working electrode to a periodic digital signal, the frequency of which is proportional to the concentration of the presence of bacterial pathogen [11].

The integrated potentiostat is composed of a potential controller and a current-to-frequency converter (CFC). The potential controller consisted of two operational amplifiers and two load transistors. The function is to control the potential difference at the interface between the solution droplet and working electrode, where an electrochemical reaction occurred. This operation is accomplished by reading the input voltage (V_{in}) and adjusting the voltage at the counter electrode

(CE), so that the potential difference between the voltages at the reference electrode (RE) and working electrode (WE) are equal to V_{in}. On the other hand, the current-to-frequency converter is consisted of two operational amplifiers, one-shot circuit, dynamic flip-flop and load transistor. The function is to convert the electrical current through the working electrode (WE) into a periodic digital signal. The amplifier is a conventional two-stage operational amplifier design with n-type differential input pair. The open-loop gain of the operational amplifiers is higher than 86 dB while the cutoff frequency is roughly 500 kHz as shown in Figure 4-7. Although these performances were not comparable with CMOS technologies, they were high enough to compose the integrated potentiostat because the electric current and operation frequency are not so high.

The trans-impedance amplifier (TIA) has fully integrated components in its feedback loop. Figure 4-8 shows the schematic of the TIA. The bias signal (V_p), the counter electrode (CE), and the digital controls are all provided externally.

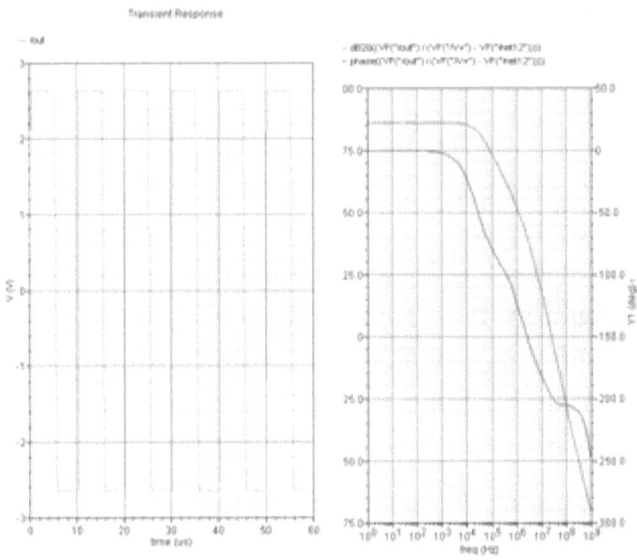

Figure 4-7   The simulation result for the TIA operation amplifier.

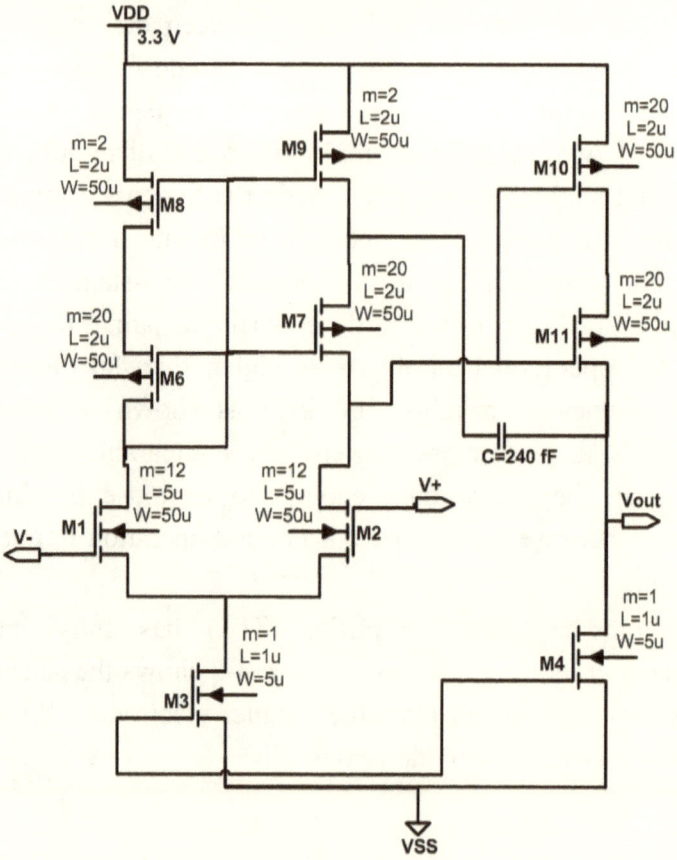

Figure 4-8   The schematic of TIA used in the first stage.

The operational amplifiers in each stage use a gain-boosted folded cascade topology, and all the transistors within the sensor (including switches) use thick-oxide I/O devices (0.35-μm minimum channel length in the process) that accommodate a maximum allowable supply of 3.3 V. Since most electroanalytical methods, with perhaps the exception of impedance spectroscopy, essentially operate at low frequency (i.e., below 100 kHz).

4.5   Microfluidic Electrochemical cell

The electrochemical cell device lies on measuring the variation in the electrical potential occurring between the electrodes in the electrolyte solution using high input impedance devices. The electrochemical cell consists of a three-electrode configuration known as counter, reference, and working electrodes. Conventionally, the electrochemical cell is fabricated using a soft photolithography technique employing semiconductor material or glass slices. The fabrication process using the soft photolithography technique was largely reported in the literature [12][13]. Figure 4-9 illustrates the basic microfluidic channel (MFC) with three inlets, an analyte, washing and micelles, and outlet.

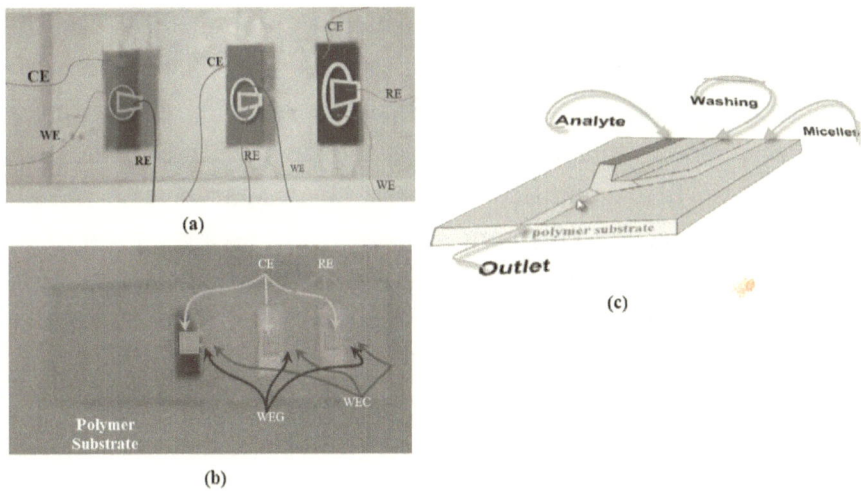

Figure 4-9   Basic Microfluidic channel with three inlets and outlet.

Recently, CMOS/MEMS technology made large contributions to the biomedical transducer through utilizing microfabrication techniques that can apply to produce a variety of geometries, i.e. sizes, shapes, that are named microelectrodes compared to conventional fabrication techniques.

Figure 4-10 shows the microfluidic channel (MFC) embedded with interdigitated microelectrode arrays (IDMA) as a sensing surface referring to the working electrode in the basic electrochemical cell structure that was previously introduced by [14][15].

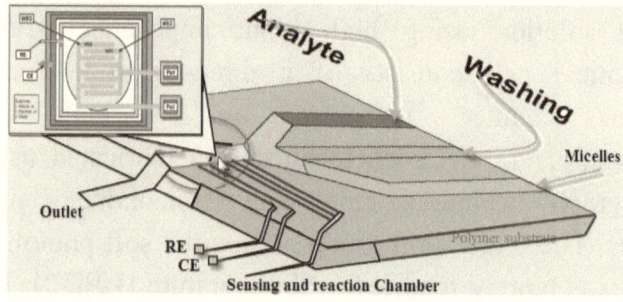

Figure 4-10 Microfluidic channel with embedded interdigitated microelectrodes array.

IDMAs are widely used particularly in biomedical and life science applications for many advantages. Besides their low cost and thus their high mass-production, IDMA offers tiny size that leads to produce a small voltage drop across the fingers which yields to a high electric filed generated. The overall design came to a novel design named as the polymeric lab on a chip laying on top of the CMOS chip with the embedded interdigitated microelectrodes array, as shown in Figure 4-11 [16]. Physically; there are two types of diffusions; linear and radical (spherical). Although the macroelectrodes suffer from the first diffusion, the IDMA takes advantage of the spherical diffusion to rapidly establish a steady-state mass transfer and a high current density value "$J = \frac{I}{A}$", resulting in the decrease of the current value as given by the equation.

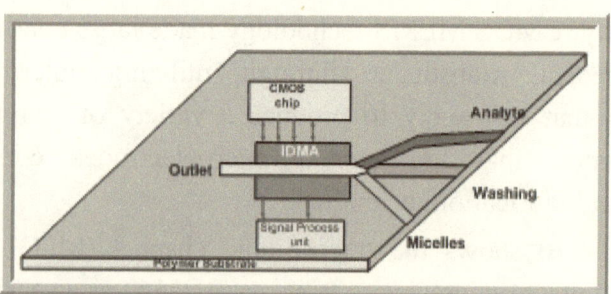

Figure 4-11 Polymeric lab on a chip on top of CMOS chips with embedded interdigitated microelectrodes array.

Due to the Faradaic process and In the light of ohm's law "$V = IR$", the voltage drop across the fingers is low. This makes the bio-transducer, including the IDMA, to work independently in the biomedical environment[17]. In the light of the Non-Faradaic process, the presence of the IDMA in the system yields to tiny capacitive displacement currents [18]. Figure 4-12 illustrates the fundamental of interdigitated microelectrode arrays.

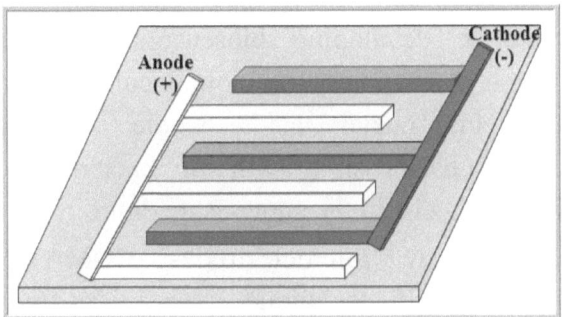

Figure 4-12 Basic Interdigitated microelectrode array (IDMA) Illustrating the anode and cathode terminals.

These electrodes are created by parallel fingers in a 100-µm length, 1 µm width and 0.5-µm spacing. The IDMA are interconnected with the aim of acquiring an anode and a cathode. In the electrochemical cell, the anode is where oxidation takes place, referring to the positive polarity contact where negative ions are enforced by applying external potential, which leads to a production of electrons as an oxidation process. On the other hand, the cathode presents the negative polarity contact, thus, the reduction takes place. [19]. The flow of the electrolyte control in the microchannel is achieved by means of a high precision syringe pump in pushing mode connected to the channel inlet. Operation in pushing mode permits introducing the nanoparticle suspension by simple pipetting into the inlet reservoir of the microfluidic chip holder. Once the microchannel is homogeneously filled, the capture and dosing of the biological cells will start. [20][21].

At that point, the flow is stopped and a current is applied to generate the local electrical field between the anode and cathode of the IDMA required for plug formation. An AC current and field is used throughout the experiments (50 Hz or 100 Hz) and the bacterial pathogen cells instantaneously align with the external field.

4.5.1 The characteristics of IDMA influences and advantages

Recently, interdigitated array microelectrodes have grown a widespread use in developing biosensors for monitoring the catalyzed reaction of enzymes, the biomolecular recognition events of specific proteins, nucleic acids, whole cells, antibodies or antibody-related substances; growth of bacterial cells, or the presence of bacterial cells in the aqueous medium.

Interdigitated array microelectrodes (IDMA) have been integrated with the EIS technique in order to miniaturize the conventional electrodes, enhance the sensitivity and use the flexibility of electrode fabrication to suit the conventional electrochemical cell format or microfluidic devices for a variety of applications in chemistry and life sciences application. This work is focused on IDMA based on the EIS technique as biosensors for their applications in pathogens detection. Some researchers elaborated on different IDMA geometries, their fabrication materials, design parameters and types of detection techniques [22][23].

The IDMA with a four-electrode configuration as shown in Figure 4-13, was fabricated on polymer or glass wafers and investigated to obtain optimal oxidation and reduction reactions [24]. The IDMA is made of proximity microbands of an array to probe chemistry taking place around the microband. The four-electrode configuration implies a working electrode constructed of a double-band system named as the generator-collector mode. The two fingers' proximity aid the diffusion fields to overlap and a mutual effect occurs in between fingers.

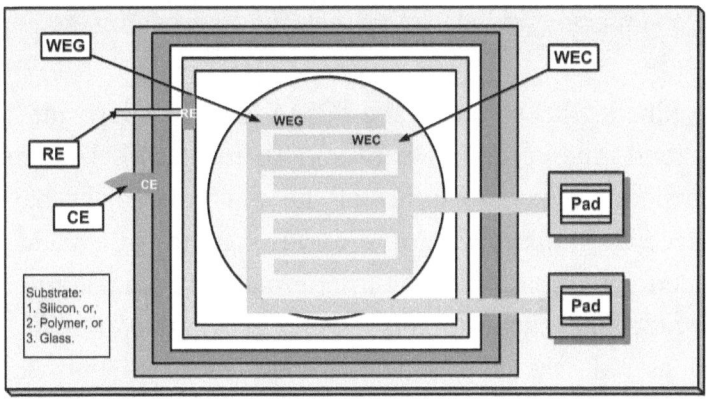

Figure 4-13 The four-electrode configuration.

The mechanism of this configuration simply lies on the generator electrode that acts as a driver producing reduction species and the collector electrode that collects the generated reduction species so a current flows as result of this process. The generation-collection mode is sensitive to the chemical stability of species reduction. The dynamic motion of the oxidation-reduction reaction has the capability for detecting and quantifying the process. In the case of insufficient time to diffuse ions to the collector, no current flow implies that no generating ions at the generator occurs, otherwise a current is recorded. Therefore, the more current is recorded, the higher sensitivity of the electrode required. The high sensitivity of this configuration comes from the feedback that occurs from the oxidation species at one finger to the oxidation species on the other finger. The feedback influence is playing an important role in the identification and quantification of chemical reactions concerning oxidation and reduction species. The generation-collection working electrode mode can be achieved using a two-finger and three-finger interfering configuration. In the three-finger configuration, the middle finger represents the generator and the adjacent fingers act as collectors. The more complicated technique can be achieved through the IDMA that is a comb built of wide series of parallel fingers. This comb is interfered with the other comb, therefore one of the combs acts as a collector and the other acts as a generator as shown in Figure 4-14.

The kinetics behaviors of the IDMA relay on the widths of the fingers and the spacing between them [25]. The principal consequences of the properties of the microelectrodes have been categorized by Stulik *et al.* [26]. A steady state for a Faradaic process is obtained very rapidly leading to improve the Faradaic-to-charging current ratio and signal-to-noise ratio. In addition, scaling up the dimensions of the electrodes allows measurements on tiny biomolecular volume.

Interdigitated microelectrodes arrays aim to enhance the signal-to-noise ratio, therefore, many researchers investigated various parameters of the IDMA [27][28]. Interesting differences between the electrode materials gold and platinum were found, which were due to the oxidization of platinum and gold during the IDMA fabrication process, where the microelectrodes of various geometries have been prepared mechanically or lithographically.

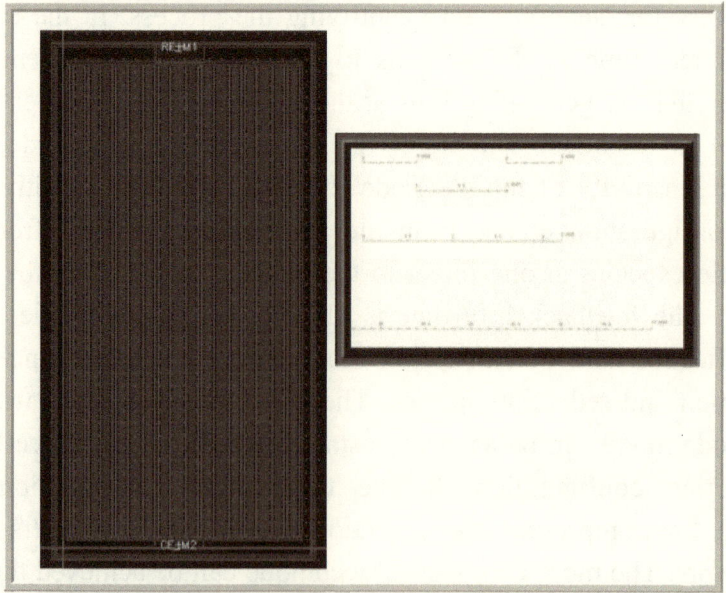

Figure 4-14 The layout of the IDMA.

It resulted in gold IDMA as being by far superior in respect to signal-to-noise ratio and overall signal magnitude to those made of platinum [29].

4.6 Electrochemical impedance spectroscopy Structure and Behavior

EIS is a rapid and powerful technique due to its capability to show thorough information straightforwardly on biorecognition-event induced capacitance and resistance, which alter at the IDMA or the substrate's surface. For instance, when antibodies bind to antigens resulting in an alteration in the impedance of the system, it makes possible the direct measurement of an electrical signal[30][31]. Physically, biological cells for their tiny volume and structure can electrically describe underprivileged conductors at low frequencies; i.e. below 10 kHz. For this reason, the effect of biological cells on the interface impedance will be insignificant; such serious issues should be resolved. In order to make the biosensors work efficiently in biomedical and life science applications, some procedures are strongly required and applied to biological systems by applying external electrical potential; current or voltage, to entirely avoid this serious obstacle. Bacteria cells grow adherently on the surface of microelectrodes. Consequently, the electrode area that is exposed for the applied electrical signal will be significantly reduced. This implies that the measured impedance, which is inversely proportional to this parameter, is increased accordingly [32]. Growing biological cells adherently is an essential and fundamental process of all biological systems where the cell-host interface detection process takes place because of cells undergoing extensive cell-cell and cell-extracellular matrix interactions [33][34]. EIS technique is integrated with IDMA; the bound cells are cultured directly on the sensing surface of the IDMA thus the overall signal that is carried out by impedance measurements lies on three features related to adherently growing cells. These features alter the number, growth and morphological behavior of the adherent cells due to the cell membranes acting as insulators [35]. It is important to note that any alters in media will result in dramatic alteration on the impedance measurement due to the permittivity changing [36][37]. The detection of biological cells using the EIS based impedance biosensors can be performed using the Non-Faradaic process in the absence of redox probes where the adherent growth of biological cells causes an alteration in the ionic structure. Therefore, the impedance in its components, both the imaginary and real parts, can be recorded and plotted using the Bode diagram [38][39].

On other hand, the EIS based impedance technique can be also performed using the Faradaic process in the presence of a redox probe. This technique mainly lies on sensing the formation of antibody-antigen immunoreactions on sensing surfaces of the IDMA through monitoring the double layer capacitance and charge-transfer resistance of electrodes-electrolyte interface. The bioreceptors; i.e. antibodies, have an important role in this process due to generating impenetrable nanoparticles that serve for an amplification strategy. This amplifies the alteration in the charge-transfer resistance because of the binding of biological cells to the sensing surface. However, the Faradaic process adds more steps for the system. As a result, a non-Faradaic process as a free-label technique is widely used due to its high ability of detecting the alterations of the electrical properties proximity surface [40].

A high density of IDMA is used as a sensing surface to detect a concentration of biological cells in a solution. Once biological cells are attached to antibodies, only one part of the biological cell is covered above the sensor surface. As soon as the IDMA is dunked in a solution, only the active area of the biological cells is exposed to the solution. The purpose of the immobilized surface of the antibodies between the electrodes is that it acts as ties that hold the biological cell in place. The more concentrations of biological cells bound to the sensing surface the more changes noted in impedance measurements in between the microbands [41]. The EIS is deployed for bacteria detection in biosensors that are based on impedance analysis of the electrical properties of biological cells when they are binding to or associated with the microelectrode array [42].

Generally, impedance measurements can be Faradaic, which is a charge-transfer process that is joint together by electrons transferring across the interface leading to the reduction or oxidation of species present at the interface [43]:

$$ox + ne \leftrightarrow Re \tag{4.6}$$

Where "Ox" is oxidation reaction and "Re" is reduction reaction. The dynamic behavior of the redox reaction can be described using the Butler-Volmer relationship:

$$i = nF[k_f C_{ox}(0) - k_b C_{Re}(0)] \tag{4.7}$$

Where F is the Faraday constant, C_{Ox}, and C_{Re} are the surface concentration, n is the number of electrons, and k_f and k_b are the potential-dependant rate constant for the oxidation and reduction reactions. The Faraday impedance depends on the reaction mechanism given by:

$$Z_f = \frac{V}{i} \tag{4.8}$$

Therefore, the total faraday impedance is [44]:

$$Z_f = \left(\frac{RT}{n^2 F^2}\right) \left(\frac{1 + \frac{k_f}{\sqrt{j\omega D_{ox}}} + \frac{k_b}{\sqrt{j\omega D_{Re}}}}{\alpha k_f C_{ox}(0) + (1+\alpha)k_b C_{Re}(0)}\right) \tag{4.9}$$

Where D_{ox} and D_{Re} are the diffusion constant for the oxidized and reduced species respectively and α is the symmetry factor. It should be emphasized that the impedance measurements are mainly used for measuring space charge capacities. They are usually performed in a frequency range of 10 kHz up to nearly 1 MHz depending on the Faraday current [45]. The double-layer capacitor (C_{dl}) devices involve mainly *non-Faradaic* accumulation of charge difference across an interface that is electrostatic rather than electrochemical [46][47]:

$$i_{nf} = \frac{dQ}{dt} \tag{4.10}$$

Where Q is the charge, t is the time, and "*I*" is the current.

Thus the structure formed in this process is called the electrical double layer; i.e. the capacitor. The impedance of a capacitance is given by:

$$Z_{dl}(w) = \frac{1}{j\omega C_{dl}} \tag{4.11}$$

Where "$J = \sqrt{-1}$" and ω is the angular frequency and C_{dl} is the double layer capacitor. The total impedance for the electrolyte/electrode interface is given by:

$$Z(\omega) = \frac{R_t}{1+j\omega R_t C_{dl}} \tag{4.12}$$

Consequently, Faradaic and non-Faradaic impedance can be categorized based on the presence or absence of any redox probe respectively. Non-Faradaic impedance is an alternative impedance technique in favor of developing biosensors for the detection of bacteria as well as cell-based sensors. The variant of the impedance signal is depending on the growth and morphology behaviors of the adherent cells' number due to the insulating effects of the cell membranes. The growth of bacteria on the electrode surface can be detected in the absence of a redox probe. For this reason, it causes a change in the ionic composition resulting in the impedance of the medium, independent of the volume of the sample, that will change simultaneously along with the bacteria concentration [50]. The measurement of the impedance results from the bacteria cells that are adherently growing on the electrode surface [51].

The microfluidic channel (MFC) incorporated with the IDMAs is used as the transducer-sensing surface that will functionalize by specific antibodies against a target bacterial pathogen strain. Interdigitated microelectrodes arrays have a lot of advantages besides their short electric field penetration depth that is capable to analyze the electrical properties of thin layers and membranes [52][53].

IDMA can be employed for detecting the presence of particular dielectric objects on the surface of electrodes [54][55]. After the sensing surface is represented by interdigitated microelectrodes that are exposed to an applied electrical field, the impedimetric detection perform to analyze and study the behavior of the biomolecular samples in the microfluidic channel. As aforementioned in section 2.2.2, the double layer capacitance (C_{dl}) in the electrolyte behaves similar to two simple parallel plates.

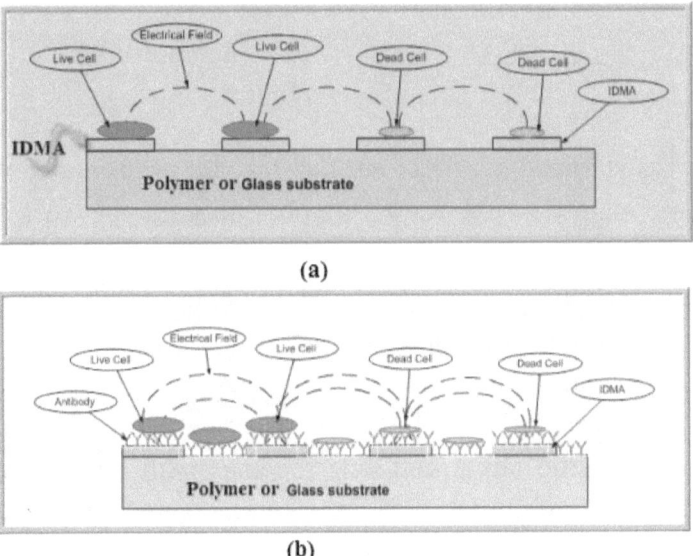

(a)

(b)

Figure 4-15 The electric field established between the fingers (a) free-label (b) Antibodies process.

For the impedimetric detection of bacterial pathogens, a suitable frequency should be selected under a specific electrical field that is applied in the presence of bacterial pathogens binding to the surface of the electrodes via the biomolecular recognition of antibodies. Therefore, the entire system will perturb and the variation will be detectable and measurable. Besides, the geometries of the electrodes and the interface gap between the electrolyte and electrode are playing a significant role in the cell performance [56]. As soon as the surface of the sensing transducer is modified by filling it with biomolecular sample as a new dielectric in between the interdigitated electrodes, there would be variation in the measured impedance. The Z_T components are the real part; Z_{Re}, which is the resistance of the solution increased and the imaginary one; Z_{Im} that decreases the double layer capacitance accordingly:

$$Z_T = Z_{Re} + Z_{Im} = R_{sol} - \frac{\frac{jR_{ct}}{\omega C_{dl}}}{R_{ct} - \frac{j}{\omega C_{dl}}} \tag{4.13}$$

$$Z_{Re} = R_{sol} + \frac{R_{ct}}{1 + (\omega R_{ct} C_{dl})^2} \tag{4.14}$$

$$Z_{Im} = -\frac{R_{ct}^2 \omega C_{dl}}{1 + (\omega R_{ct} C_{dl})^2} \tag{4.15}$$

EIS based impedimetric biosensors that are incorporated with the IDMA are mainly in use due to the proximity gap between fingers. This leads to a generated strong electrical field between the fingers therefore yielding a transducer with high performance. The mechanism of this technique depends on the generated electrical field, where it starts from one side and ends on the other side of the IDMA as shown in Figure 4-15. The electrical field is spreading in the gap where the target cell acts together with the bioreceptors, which are antibodies used for the label process creating a disturbance of the generated electric field. The group of Gijs [57] overcomes the ionic media that is the major disadvantage in such a method due to the pre-dominant electrical distribution resistance of the electrolyte.

In fact, the improvement lies on the optimization of the washing step subsequent to the target hybridization with the purpose of getting rid of all the ions from the electrolyte [58].

In the presence of the electrical field, the biomolecular particles will align and get denser causing the situation to differ from before, where the magnitude of the alteration in the cell constant significantly relies on both the size and area of the sensing surface covered by biomolecular particles, as shown in Figure 4-16. The label-free and direct electrical detection of tiny biomolecular particles and proteins is possible by their intrinsic charges using biofunction ion-sensitive technique. The biofunctionalization of the sensing surfaces coated with gold can be performed with BSA.

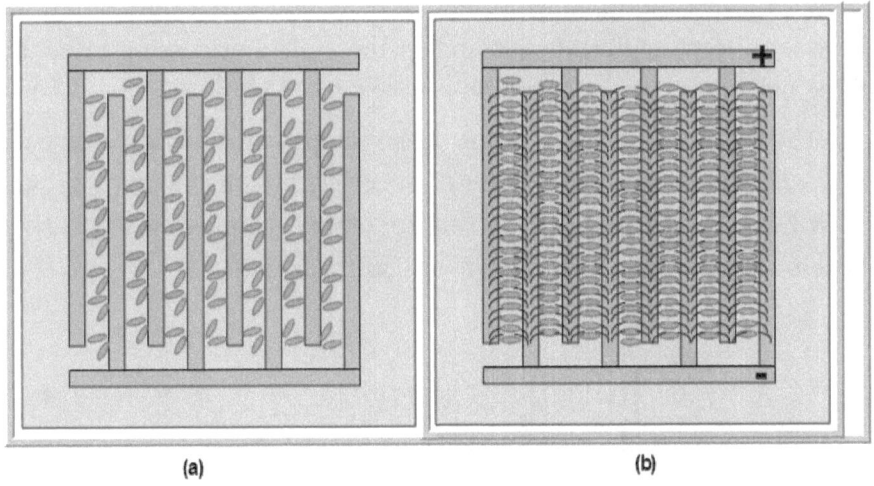

(a) (b)

Figure 4-16 The sensing surface covered by bacterial pathogen (a) before and (b) after applying electrical field.

To achieve the biofunctionalization, a specific protocol should be applied [59]. The integrated system as described here will have an enormous potential to concentrate and enhance bacterial capture from samples.

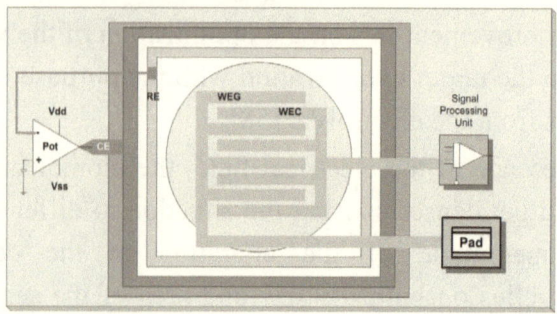

Figure 4-17 The architecture of the electrochemical biosensors.

This integration should improve the detection limit by several orders of magnitude, shorten the analysis and reduce non-specific detection events. Figure 4-17 illustrates the schematic detection setup. In this setup, a four-electrode configuration is placed in between the potentiostat unit and in the signal-processing unit, the three units build up the entire biosensor CMOS chip.

The electrode surfaces of the sensor chips will functionalize with the recognition receptors as a specific binding agent. Figure 4-18shows the layout of the entire electrochemical CMOS chip beside the schematic of the entire system.

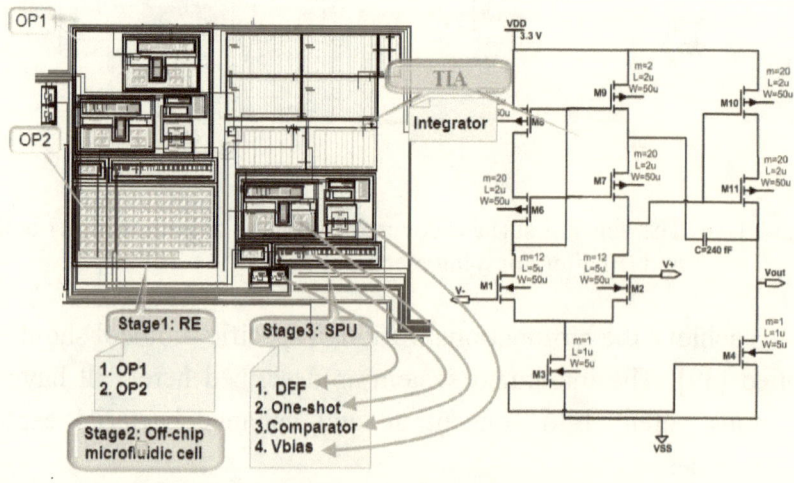

Figure 4-18 (a) The layout of the EIS CMOS chip, (b) The schematic of TIA.

The detection system approach has the following protocol that should be applied for achieving the mission of this transducer successfully; captured biological cells are introduced over the array containing the electrodes coated with the specific recognition elements. As soon as the electrical field is applied to the captured analytes, bacterial pathogens for instance, on the sensor surface, the impedance as a response of the sensor will change due to the added bacteria that is captured by a cytogenetic technique [60]. The cytogenetic technique is one of the methodologies of genetics that covers the configuration and behavior of the biological cell, especially the chromosomes. Therefore, it is considered as a dominant approach for detecting RNA or DNA sequences in cells, tissues, and tumors. Conjugate fluorophores that are used as labels with *in-situ* hybridization has come to be known as fluorescent *in-situ* hybridization (FISH) that is used to detect and confine the presence or absence of specific DNA sequences on chromosomes and mRNA contained by tissues accordingly [61].

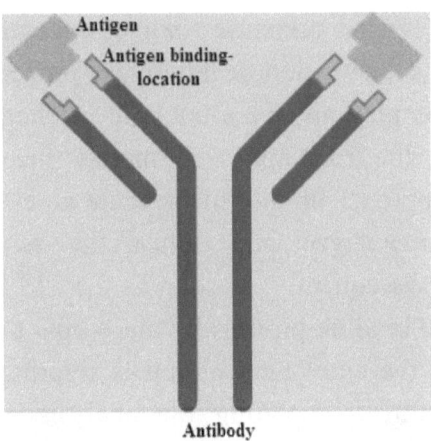

Figure 4-19 Immunoglobulin attaches to a unique antigen.

The reporter gene signal can be readily amplified by fluorophore-tagged immunoglobulin (Ig) that are bound to the dye molecule where each immunoglobulin binds to a unique antigen as shown in

Figure 4-19. By measuring the impedance; as a biosensor response, which has bound onto the sensing surface, the rapid detection and quantitation of the presence of the specific biological cell is allowed.

4.7 Equivalent Circuit modeling of the Immunosensor System

Electrochemical impedance spectroscopy (EIS) is discussed and considered as a powerful bioanalytical and clinical approach where the frequency dependence of the biosensor response can be readily carried out. To investigate and understand the potential differences at phase boundaries in biological and physiological processes, the electrical polarization and the charge-exchange process is performed by using electrochemistry technique [62]. The nature of the biological cells growth and its environmental variations has a drawback that leads to insufficient and inaccurate information to describe the physical and chemical characteristics of the biosensor. It is essential and beneficial to understand these characteristics in order to optimize the sensor response. Some uncontrolled parameters might occur during incubation or laboratory procedures; preparation and washing steps play an important role in altering the biosensor response making the EIS approach merely incomplete. For that reason, the EIS approach should incorporate an electrical equivalent circuit model to analyze and adjust the assorted parameters concerned [63]. Consequently, as soon as the EIS approach is doing its job through the binding process by measuring the frequency band over a shot time, the equivalent circuit is figuring out the changes caused by drift thus completing the analysis of the impedance behavior of the biosensor [64].

The physical foundation of the impedance alterations can be identified using the response of the interface with equivalent circuit models. Generally, a collection of interfaces, which are represented as an electrochemical microfluidic cell, readily characterizes its performance by an equivalent circuit model built of resistors and capacitors that pass current with the same amplitude and phase angle. The real electrochemical cell behaves after applying external potential. Randles proposed the basic model in electrochemistry, as shown in Figure 4-20. In Randle's equivalent circuit, each of the four circuit elements represents a separate and clearly identifiable physical phenomenon. These elements are; resistance R_{sol} for the electrolyte resistance, capacitance C_{dl}, which represents the electrical double layer at the electrode/solution interface for the interfacial combination of electronic and ionic charges, and the resistance R_{ct} as a byproduct of the electrochemical reactions happening at the interface, which is a quantity of charge leaking across the double layer [65]. For that reason the charge transfer resistance, R_{ct} is shown on the circuit to represent this charge leakage, and the diffusion of ions to the interface from the bulk of the electrolyte causes impedance that is well-known as Warburg impedance. Z_W. Z_W represents the impedance of diffusion of the contributors in the Faradaic processes towards and from the interface.

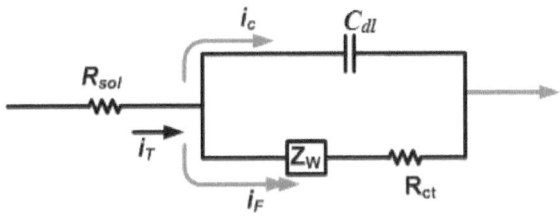

Figure 4-20 Randles equivalent electrical circuit model.

The Warburg impedance cannot be simply observed physically at lower frequencies less than 1 kHz. It is covered by the inverse of the sampling period due to the slow electron-transfer kinetics. In the absence of the Warburg impedance, the shape of the impedance, Nyquist plot Z_{Im} vs. Z_{Re}, does not look good except when a constant phase element (C_{PE}) is added to the model [66]. The C_{PE} is an admittance that can be characterized as $Y_{CPE} = Y_0 (j\omega)^\alpha$ where Y_0 and α are the parameters of C_{PE}, α is the parameter that is more likely to define the nature of this quantity sites within the range $-1 \leq \alpha \leq 1$ and Y_{CPE} ends at the admittance when $\alpha = 1$ hence $Y_{CPE} = j\omega C_{dl}$ where C_{dl} is the double layer capacitance. In the impedance, the electrochemical microfluidic channel can be measured by [67]:

$$Z_T = R_s + \left[\frac{1}{R_{ct}} + Y_{CPE}\right]^{-1} \qquad (4.16)$$

In the simple form of the equivalent circuit, three elements are essential to carry out the linear diffusion impedance. The element R_s refers to the solution electrical behavior. The capacitor C_{dl} models the double-layer, where the electrical double-layer sometimes is represented by a constant-phase element (C_{PE}) and a parallel resistance R_{dl} [68]. The resistance R_{ct} relates to the charge transfer. Z_w is the Warburg impedance related to the mass transfer. The last constant phase element is modeling the low frequency behavior of the cell. Others defined the capacitance of the electrochemical double layer in series with the native silicon-oxide layer capacitance, which is modeled in the electrical equivalent circuit as a C_{PE}. It comprises deviation from the ideal behavior of a capacitor and it occurs at low frequencies [69]. Robert Levie [70] commented on the most popular model used in electrochemical analysis considering Randles' equivalent circuit, and proved that it is not reasonable and that it is exception rather than the rule. Consequently, the equivalent circuits' models are unsuccessfully right to represent such subtleties. Some arrangements with the double-layer capacitance; C_{dl} as a frequency-dependent constant-phase element [C_{PE}] is given by [70]:

$$CPE = Y_0 \, (j\omega)^{-\alpha} \qquad (4.17)$$

The C_{PE} element is convenient for the flattened semicircle, which initiates from noticeable non-capacitive reactance properties. The C_{PE} element appears at low frequencies and it is modeled as a C_{PE} to account for deviations from the ideal behavior of a capacitor [71][72]. Note that the resistance associated to the silicon substrate; R_{sub} and the stray capacitance of the polysilicon electrodes to the silicon substrate through the silicon oxide-insulating layer C_{sub} have almost no influence on the impedance measurement. Since R_{Si} and C_{subs} are substrate parameters and constant among all biosensors, they can be ignored and eliminated from the equivalent circuit.

The electrochemical impedance spectroscopy measurements of the total microfluidic cell or microelectrode impedance as a function of frequency (ω) and techniques can be willingly taken out of the Faradaic impedance; Z_f, the solution resistance; R_{sol}, and the double-layer capacitance; C_{dl} from direct measurements plots; such as Nyquist and bode plots. Nyquist plots can be acquired from and compared to equivalent circuit models that are built up of different components based on the appropriate equations on behalf of the rates of the various methods and their contributions to the current.

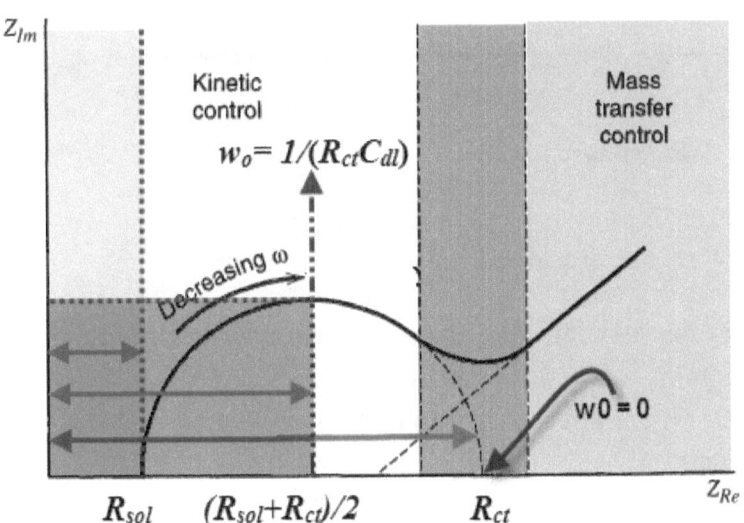

Figure 4-21 The general schematic drawing of Nyquist plot for an EIS.

Figure 4-21 shows the general Nyquist plot. On the other hand, such equivalent circuits are inclusive, so it is hard to select the form or structure of the equivalent circuit from the processes involved in the reaction scheme. In a complex reaction method, simple circuit models such as Randles' model is incorrect and insufficient for deliberate admittance or impedance measurements. Because of some significant parameters in the AC response in the EIS that should be considered such as the electrode surface roughness and heterogeneity [73] and as long as no experimental pledge is seen in the horizon, the equivalent circuit model cannot mirror the performance of the system.

For the all these reasons; the measurement of the impedance based on the standard equivalent circuit as shown in Figure 4-20 should go further in depth. Consequently, the measurement can be performed either separately or altogether but the latter is more preferable and applicable for varies of frequencies and for the Faradaic impedance. The equivalent circuit is shown in Figure 4-22.

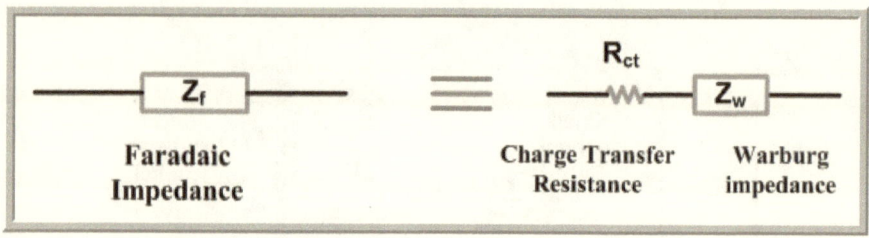

Figure 4-22 Faradaic impedance and its equivalent.

For non-Faradaic impedance, the equivalent circuit is shown in Figure 4-23. Using this approach makes it easier and the parameters R_{sol}, R_{ct}, C_d are directly determined, thus the total impedance Z_T can be written as:

$$Z_T(\omega) = Z_1 + \frac{Z_2 Z_3}{Z_2 Z_3} \tag{4.18}$$

Where; $Z_1 = R_{sol}$, $Z_2 = -\frac{j}{\omega C_{dl}}$, and $Z_3 = R_{ct}$. The electrochemical impedance spectroscopic approach deals with the variation of total impedance in the complex plane as represented by Nyquist plots. The total impedance (Z_T) of the electrochemical cell can be described in two parts, real and imaginary parts [74]. Both parts of the impedance; Z_{Re} and Z_{Im} should be measured and matched with the experiments protocols that are defined as follow:

$$Z_{Re} = R_{SOL} + \frac{R_{ct}+\sigma\omega^{-1/2}}{(C_{dl}\sigma\omega^{1/2}+1)^2+\omega^2 C_{dl}^2(R_{ct}+\sigma\omega^{-1/2})^2} \qquad (4.19)$$

$$Z_{Im} = \frac{\omega C_{dl}(R_{ct}+\sigma\omega^{-1/2})^2+\sigma\omega^{-1/2}(C_{dl}\sigma\omega^{1/2}+1)}{(C_{dl}\sigma\omega^{1/2}+1)^2+\omega^2 C_{dl}^2(R_{ct}+\sigma\omega^{-1/2})^2} \qquad (4.20)$$

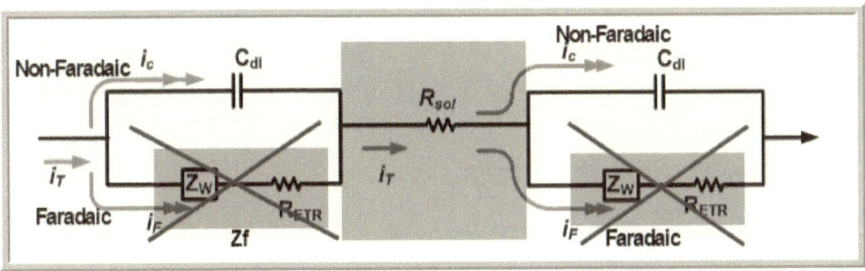

Figure 4-23 Non-Faradaic equivalent circuit model.

The useful chemical data can be extracted by drawing Z_{Im} vs. Z_{Re} over a range of frequencies; from low 10 Hz to 1 kHz to high frequency 50 kHz up to 1 MHz. For low frequency; "$\omega \to 0$" the above equations lead to the following equations:

$$Z_{Re} = R_{SOL} + R_{ct} + \sigma\omega^{-1/2} \qquad (4.21)$$

$$Z_{Im} = \sigma\omega^{-1/2}(C_{dl}\sigma\omega^{1/2} + 1) \qquad (4.22)$$

Solving these two equations with respect to ω yields:

$$Z_{Im} = Z_{Re} - R_{SOL} - R_{ct} + 2\sigma^2 C_{dl} \qquad (4.23)$$

This means that the relation between the two parts is linear and the slop is equal to unity. In addition, the two parts of the impedance are still frequency dependent but excluding the Warburg impedance variable. Therefore, in low frequency, the total impedance Z_T is a function of a diffusion-controlled process. As soon as the frequency rises, it enters the high regime; hence, the total impedance no longer depends on Z_w but heavily depends on parameters R_{ct} and C_{dl}. In the high frequency regime "$\omega \gg 0$"; the Warburg impedance is abandoned due to the time scale that is so short, it is not capable to back up the diffusion to dynamically operate the current.

The total impedance is fully dependant on the charge-transfer resistance; $R_{ct} = \dfrac{RT}{nFi_0}$ and the double-layer capacitance; C_{dl} where Z_w is negligible. Therefore, the two parts of the total impedance yield:

$$Z_{Re} = R_{SOL} + \frac{R_{ct}}{1+\omega^2 C_{dl}^2 R_{ct}^2} \tag{4.24}$$

$$Z_{Im} = \frac{\omega C_{dl} R_{ct}^2}{1+\omega^2 C_{dl}^2 R_{ct}^2} \tag{4.25}$$

Solving these two equations with respect to ω yields:

$$\left(Z_{Re} - R_{SOL} + \frac{R_{ct}}{2}\right)^2 + Z_{Im}^{\ 2} = \left(\frac{R_{ct}}{2}\right)^2 \tag{4.26}$$

The above result leads to a semicircle plot with radius; $r = \dfrac{R_{ct}}{2}$ and its origin at ($Z_{Im} = 0$, $Z_{Re} = R_{SOL} + \dfrac{R_{ct}}{2}$) as illustrated in Figure 4-21.:

$$\sigma = \frac{RT}{n^2 F^2 A \sqrt{2}} \left(\frac{1}{D_{Ox}^{1/2} C_{Ox}^*} + \frac{1}{D_{Re}^{1/2} C_{RE}^*}\right) \tag{4.27}$$

$$R_{ct} = \frac{RT}{nFi_0} \tag{4.28}$$

$$C_{dl} = \frac{\varepsilon_0 \epsilon_i A}{d_i} \tag{4.29}$$

Where σ is quantitatively predictable from the constants of the experiment; C_{Ox}^* and C_{Re}^* are the surface concentrations, F is the Faraday constant, T is the temperature in Kelvin, R is the Boltzmann constant, A is the exposed area and n is the number of electrons. Increasing the thickness of the surface layer causes significant decrease in the double layer capacitance constant phase element relating to the above equation where ε_0 is the vacuum dielectric constant; 8.85 x 10^{14} F/cm^2, ε_i is the dielectric constant of the layer i and A is the area of the surface.

So far, the total impedance measurement somehow is still in standard form. In practice and more accurate system the situation is more complex and the actual plot of the impedance in the complex plane will unite the two limiting features; mass-transfer and kinetic control regions. A Nyquist plot is so essential for the electrochemical system impedance where the two limiting feature regions are defined at low and high frequencies, which are the mass-transfer and kinetic control regions, respectively. Among the entire parameters of the total impedance, the key that controls the process is the charge-transfer resistance, R_{ct} incorporated with the Warburg impedance as a function of "σ". The semicircular region does not look perfect due the entire behavior of the system where the mass transfer is a significant factor. The charge-transfer resistance is dominant as long as the chemical system is kinetically slow. On the other hand, the charge-transfer resistance, R_{ct} might be slightly small by comparison to the solution resistance and the Warburg impedance over nearly the completely available range of "σ".

The equivalent circuit models were modified from the basic model that was proposed by Randles as shown on Figure 4-20. An electrical equivalent circuit is anticipated to analyze a variety of parameters involved in the impedance measurement of the target bacteria using the microfluidic channel (MFC) embedded with IDMA to improve the biosensor sensitivity [75]. Impedance measurements are often fit and adjusted to the equivalent circuit model that matches the requirement of each project individually. In electrochemical cell analysis, there are mostly a few parameters of concern to be detected based upon the range of frequency and the biological sample. The electrochemical system has Faradaic Z_f and non-Faradaic; R_{sol} and C_{dl}, impedances. The main two components in the plot, C_{dl} and R_{ct}, depend on the dielectric and insulating characteristics at the electrode/electrolyte interface. Where the double-layer capacitance C_{dl} depends on the dielectric permittivity established by the double-charged layer molecules, "ϵ_{dl}", where the dielectric constant of the vacuum is "$\varepsilon_0 = 8.85 \times 10^{-12}\, Fm^{-1}$". The effective dielectric constant of the layer separating the ionic charges is "ε_ρ", A is the electrode surface area and d is the thickness of the separating layer given by:

$$C_{dl} = \frac{\epsilon_{dl}A}{d} \;\;\rightarrow\; \epsilon_{dl} = \varepsilon_0\epsilon_\rho \qquad (4.30)$$

The double-layer capacitance, C_{dl}, can be calculated as a sum of a constant capacitance of an unmodified electrode; i.e. Au electrode, $C_{ue} \approx 40\ to\ 60\ \mu F\ cm^{-2}$, relying on the applied voltage [76], and a variable capacitance initiated from the electrode surface modifier, C_{me}, is connected as a series elements [77]

$$C_{dl} = \frac{C_{ue}C_{me}}{C_{ue}+C_{me}} \qquad (4.31)$$

In case the surface is unsmooth, the constant phase element C_{PE} is used instead of C_{dl}. The charge-transfer resistance, R_{ct}, has power over the electron transfer kinetics of the redox probe at the electrode interface. As long as the insulating modifier on the electrode is predicted to slow down the interfacial charge-transfer kinetics, then increasing the charge-transfer resistance must be done accordingly. The electron transfer resistance is determined in a similar way to the capacitance elements with respect to the unmodified electrode resistance R_{ue}, the variable charge-transfer resistance R_{me} established by the modifier and the charge-transfer resistance at the electrode that can be described in a series form and given by [77]:

$$R_{ct} = R_{ue} + R_{me} \qquad (4.32)$$

Recalling the main shape of the Faradaic impedance spectrum; Figure 4-22, Nyquist plot consists of a semicircle segment pursued by a straight line. The semicircle segment is experiential at higher frequencies with respect to the charge-transfer-limited process, while the linear part is distinguished by the lower frequency range. It represents the dispersion limited electrochemical process. The impedance spectrum can be exploited with respect for the process speed. For rapid charge transfer processes, the impedance shape can disperse to the linear part, while for a slower charge-transfer process the shape expands only in a large semicircle region. The impedance spectrum is a powerful tool to analyze and study the charge-transfer kinetics and the diffusional characteristics as well. As shown in Figure 4-21, the semicircle diameter refers to the charge-transfer resistance, R_{ct}. At high frequencies "$\omega \to \infty$" the semicircle yields an intercept with the Z_{re}-axis that refers to the solution resistance, R_{sol}. At low frequency "$\omega \to 0$" the semicircle yields an intercept correspond to $R_{sol} + R_{ct}$, where the resonance frequency is equal to "$\omega_0 = (C_{dl}R_{ct})^{-1}$" [78].

The Electrochemical analytical process can be more significant if the impedance measurements are performed with a range of frequencies "$10^{-3} < f < 10^5\ Hz$". In such condition, the interfacial properties of the modified electrodes mostly control the electrochemical process. The applied frequency is the main controller over the impedance measurements. Low frequencies less than 10^{-3} Hz result in an impedance value calculated by the DC-conductivity of the electrolyte solution, while for frequencies greater than 10^5 Hz more parameters get significant and affect the impedance spectrum as well.

Theoretically, the microfluidic cell with the three-electrode system can be treated as mentioned before; using the electrical equivalent circuit that is mainly constructed from the electrolyte solution resistance (R_{sol}), Faradaic impedance (Z_f), and double layer capacitance (C_{dl}). If there is no electrochemical reaction on the electrode surface, the Faradaic path Z_f is inactive and only the non-Faradaic impedance is operative [79]. In such a case, the equivalent circuit can be simplified as a serial combination of the electrolyte solution resistance and the double layer capacitance, which will form the total impedance (Z_T) of the system as shown in Figure 4-21. The following equations are valid and may apply:

$$\frac{1}{Z_T} = \frac{1}{Z'} + \frac{1}{Z''} \tag{4.33}$$

$$|Z'| = \sqrt{R_s^2 + \frac{1}{(\pi f C_{dl})^2}} \tag{4.34}$$

$$|Z''| = \sqrt{\frac{1}{(\pi f C_{dl})^2}} \tag{4.35}$$

For low frequencies (less than 10 kHz) the regime is capacitive dominant in which the electrode impedance could be detected and represented by the double layer capacitance and became the main source that is contributed to the total impedance. This arrangement makes the impedance value very high, where R_{sol} is insignificant. As soon as it is the high frequency range (greater than 10 kHz), the regime becomes resistive dominant due to the conduction of ions and the only contribution to the total impedance is the electrolyte resistance that is independent of the frequency and the double layer capacitance is insignificant [80]. For that reason, the growth of pathogens could be detected by the impedance measurement due to the variation in the double layer of the electrode and in the biological environment executed over a range of frequencies. In the light of what is aforementioned about the behavior of the impedance measurements, it is clearly noted that low frequency impedance (less than 10 kHz) can provide the information of the double layer capacitance of the electrode, while high frequency impedance (greater than 10 kHz) can collect the information about the electrolyte resistance. Consequently, the impedance measurement can be categorized based on what is targeted. If the biological environment is to be considered then high frequencies should be used. Otherwise, if the double layer of the electrode is to be considered then low frequencies should be used. Therefore, the impedance measurement is a powerful tool that should be used to monitor and detect the bacteria growth over a range of frequencies by watching and recording the behavior of either the double layer of the electrode or the biological environment [81]. Theoretically, the data of the electrochemical impedance spectra can be simulated with an equivalent circuit of the system for the detection of biological cells based on the general electronic equivalent model of an electrochemical cell incorporated with the behavior of the IDMA [82], as shown in Figure 4-24. Consequently, the impedance spectrum can be categorized in three separate regions corresponding to the three main elements in the equivalent circuit; the double layer capacitance, the bulk medium resistance and the dielectric capacitance of the medium based on the frequency range of the applied signal. Figure 4-24 illustrates that the Faradaic current (i_f) flows through the serial elements (R_{ETR} and Z_w) and the non-Faradaic current (i_c) flows through the double capacitance C_{dl}. The sum represents the total current that generates through the sensing surface. The total currents from the two branches will flow through the solution represented by the solution resistance R_{sol} that is plugged in series into the equivalent circuit. The components of the Faradaic components as shown in Figure 4-22 are not ideal because they are fully dependent on frequency where the components of the non-Faradaic as shown in Figure 4-23 are almost ideal circuit elements [83].

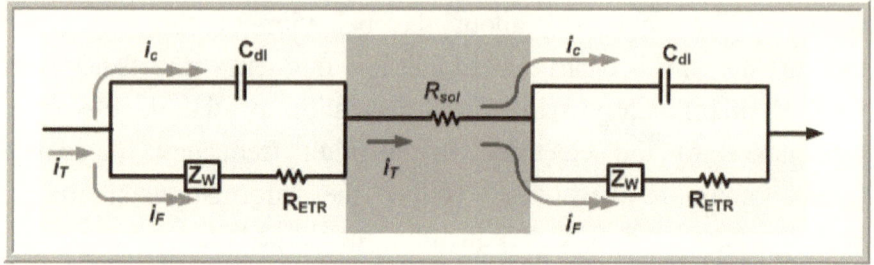

Figure 4-24 The equivalent circuit models for microelectrode array.

The first regime refers to the double layer influence at low frequency range from 10 Hz to approximately 1 kHz, the double layer capacitance of the electrodes dominates the total impedance spectra. The second regime refers to the conductivity of the ions in the medium and the bulk medium resistance over a range of frequency from 1 Hz to 50 kHz. The regime refers to the dielectric capacitance of the medium, as long as the frequency is greater than 50 kHz, then the dielectric region is dominant. At low frequency range, the double layer capacitance only dominates the impedance, while at high frequency range, the dielectric capacitance is dominant [84][85].

Algorithms analysis for electrochemical fluidic cell has been performed using potentiodynamic electrochemical impedance spectroscopy (PDEIS). PDEIS is the system for resourceful characterization of electrochemical scheme. The EIS spectrum analyzer is a standalone program for analysis and simulation of impedance spectra. Figure 4-25 shows the impedance measurements using PDEIS analyze for R_{sol} =20 Ω, R_{ct} =120 Ω, Z_w =50 Ω/s$^{1/2}$ in frequency range from 1 to 1kHz where PDEIS acquires changeable frequency responses in alternating current and a potentiodynamic DC voltammogram in the same potential scan, by probing the electrochemical interface with streams of mutually coordinated wavelets.

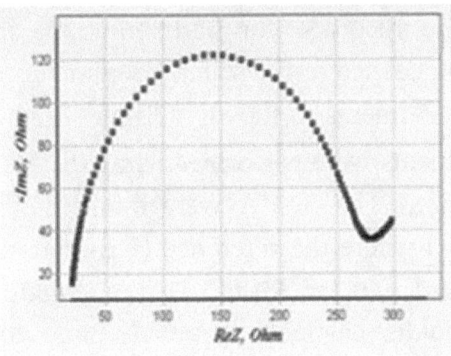

Figure 4-25 Impedance measurements using PDEIS software.

4.8 Experimental Setup and EIS on MLoC System Validation

4.8.1 Impedance measurements

The designed transducer incorporated with the MCF embedded with the IDMA is electrically characterized in deionized water as a standard solution, control sensing, and two other samples of blood and urine as surface sensing at a range of concentrations as shown in Figure 4-26.

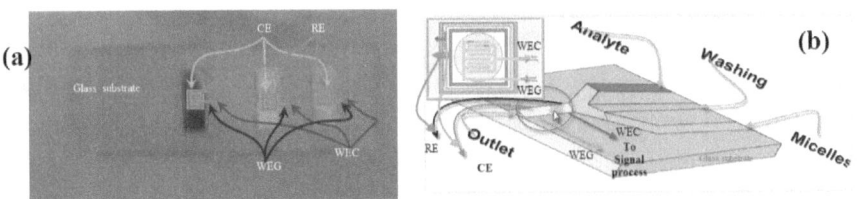

Figure 4-26 The microfluidic channel incorporates IDMA along with schematic.

The impedimetric measurements were performed at 50 mV with the frequency range 20 Hz to 1MHz. Once the system is stabilized, the solution is inserted into the MCF channel using a high precision syringe pump. The impedance measurements from low to high concentrations are recorded for both solutions individually. The analysis of the impedance response has been matched to the modified equivalent circuit elements as shown in Figure 4-24.

EIS measurements were performed using the MLoC system as an impedance analyzer. The IDMA were dunk in PBS solution as a sensing part (WE) where the reference (RE) and counter electrodes (CE) were plugged into the MLoC system. Figure 4-27 shows the different microfluidic channels that were used for validating the MLoC system.

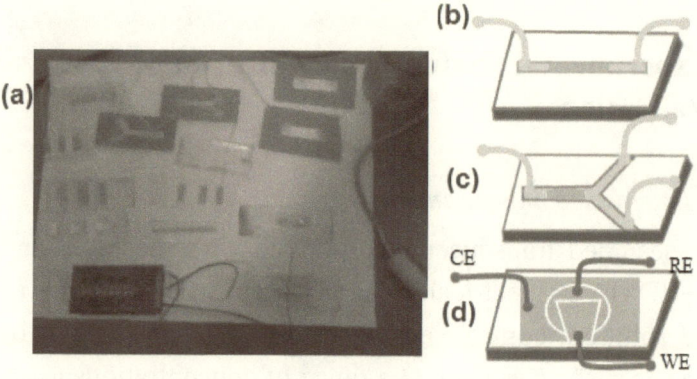

Figure 4-27 Microfluidic channels in different designs.

The experiment was performed using small AC potential within a range of frequency from 1 Hz to 100 kHz. Figure 4-28 shows the experimental setup that runs the impedance measurements. Appendix B shows more details. The state-of-the-art impedance measurements employ a frequency response analyzer that produces a sequence of alternate current of a range of frequencies. Superimposed with a DC bias current, the current is then applied to the EIS system yielding AC current measurements at each selected frequency. Afterwards, the impedance measurements were then analyzed from the excitation function. The results of the process can be recorded and drawn using Nyquist plot, imaginary impedance vs. real impedance.

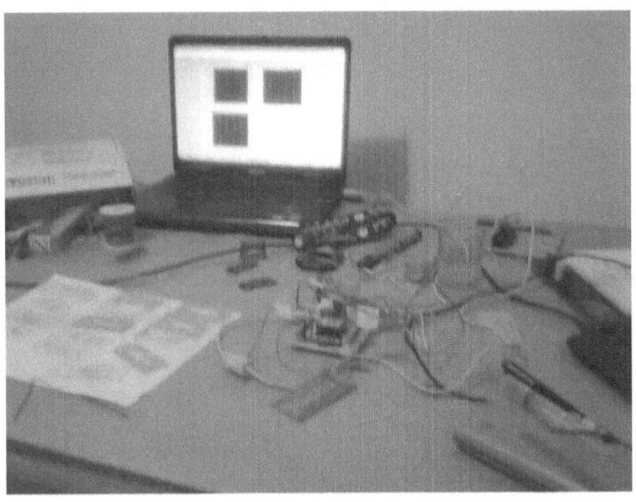

Figure 4-28 The experimental setup for impedance measurements.

The modifications on the electrode surface during the immobilization of antibodies onto the interdigitated microelectrodes array surface caused some variation mainly on the charge-transfer resistance. The changes are due to the antibody protein layer on the electrode surface that established a charge-transfer barrier and the variation increases because of the binding of biological cells on the antibody-immobilized microelectrode surface. The double layer capacitance shows variation for the immobilization of antibodies. In the medium resistance side, the binding biological cells do affect the interface resistance in the microelectrode system by creating resistance along with the medium one causing a little bit of difference from the original value of R_{sol}. The charge-transfer resistance in the semiconductor electrolyte interface can be carried out readily through a Nyquist diagram of the electrochemical impedance spectrum. The behavior of the system is tested using three different biological samples shown in Figure 4-29. Generally, the impedance spectrum has two parts a semicircle and a linear line. The semicircle part stands for the charge-transfer process with a diameter equal to the charge-transfer resistance. The linear part stands for diffusion process.

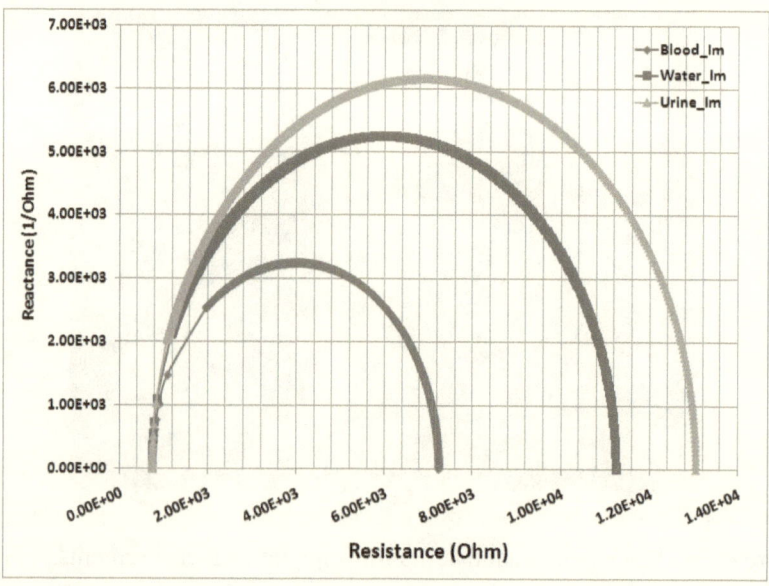

Figure 4-29 The behavior of the system after applying the three samples using Nyquist diagram.

The diameter of the semicircle represents the electron-transfer resistance at the electrode surface. The electrochemical impedance spectroscopy measurements without any amplification shows useful results for the convenience of the IDMA that are used as working electrodes for the detection of bacterial cells bound to its surface. As long as the antibody is spontaneously adsorbed due to the immobilization protocol onto the surface of microelectrodes after coating it by gold, the change in the electrochemical characteristics happened during the binding of the specific antigen. The charge-transfer resistance (R_{ct}) can be figured out from the semicircle in the Nyquist plot that is increased due to the formation of the stable antigen-antibody complex.

4.9 Summary

Electrochemical-based biosensors are specifically designed, fabricated, and experimentally validated for realizing a new generation of multi-labs-on-a-single-chip (MLoC) system. The synbook of the electrochemical biosensing with the IDMA biosensor is considered as a part out of four biosensors on the MLoC chip that worked successfully and provided enhancements in the current generation potentiostat system to impart robustness and improve the system performance when compared to the previous generations. Attributable to its compact design, multiplex capability, low cost, selective, and sensitive method, the integrated EIS is considered as a powerful tool for the detection process in medical diagnosis. This work shows how engineering fields, physics, MEMS, bioelectrochemistry, and biology are combined at VLSI by replacing the separation between immunosensors and bioreceptors with an integrative approach through utilizing CMOS based biosensing. This work is focused on the interaction between the biosensors and the matching transducer surface nano-architectures with special focus on electronic sensing. IDMA technology has a potential integrated within the microfluidic channel (MFC) for biomedical and life sciences applications and it is the main valuable outcome along with the achievement of the miniaturization of biosensors that improves the transducer's sensitivity and selectivity. Presently, EIS incorporated with IDMA based on immunosensors are introduced as solutions for point-of-care diagnosis due to the direct electronic detection that is straightforwardly scalable and integerable into the CMOS technology process. In the light of the definition of originality aforementioned in "*section* 1.4", the EIS techniques fill in the first category where the ideas have been previously published. The design in the literature made of a die within 2.25 × 2.25 mm using BiCMOS technology 1.2 μm, and power supply -2V, +7V but the tools for MLoC system are definitely different. In this design, the technology that used is CMOSP35, the area of the overall size of the CMOS potentiostat chip sites is 500 μm by 380.6 μm, and power supply is 3.3V. Furthermore, all of its stages implemented on-chip includes voltage controller and signal-processing unit along with their associating capacitors and resistors.

4.10 References

[1]   Lorenz, W.; Schulze, K. D. "Application of transform-impedance spectrometry", Journal of Electroanalytical Chemistry, 65(1), 141-153, 1975.

[2]   Dorothee Grieshaber, Robert MacKenzie, Janos Voros, Erik Reimhult, "Electrochemical Biosensors-Sensor Principles and Architectures", Sensors, 8, 1400-1458, 2008.

[3]   Arjang Hassibi, Thomas H. Lee, "A Programmable 0.18-μm CMOS Electrochemical Sensor Microarray for Biomolecular Detection", IEEE Sensors Journal, Vol. 6, No. 6, December 2006.

[4]   Peter M. Levine, Ping Gong, Rastislav Levicky, Kenneth L. Shepard, "Active CMOS Sensor Array for Electrochemical Biomolecular Detection", IEEE Journal Of Solid-State Circuits, Vol. 43, No. 8, 1859, August 2008.

[5]   Peter M. Levine, Ping Gong, Rastislav Levicky, Kenneth L. Shepard, "Real-time, multiplexed electrochemical DNA detection using an active complementary metal-oxide-semiconductor biosensor array with integrated sensor electronics", Biosensors and Bioelectronics, 2008.

[6]   Omowunmi A. Sadik, Austin O. Aluoch, Ailing Zhou, "Status of biomolecular recognition using electrochemical techniques", Biosensors and Bioelectronics, Volume 24, Issue 9, Pages 2749-2765, 15 May 2009.

[7]   Mutsumi Kimura, Hitoshi Fukushima, Yuki Sagawa, Koushi Setsu, "An Integrated Potentiostat with an Electrochemical Cell Using Thin-Film Transistors" IEEE Transactions On Electron Devices, Vol. 56, No. 9, September 2009.

[8]   Allen J. Bard, Larry R. Faulkner, "Electrochemical methods fundamentals and applications", New York: JohnWiley & Sons, 1980, pp. 563-567, 1980.

[9]   J. M. H. King, P. M. DiGrazia, B. Applegate, R. Burlage, J. Sanseverino, P. Dunbar, F. Larimer, G. S. Sayler, "Rapid, Sensitive Bioluminescent Reporter Technology for Naphthalene Exposure and Biodegradation", AAA Science, Vol. 249. no. 4970, pp. 778-781, 17 August 1990.

[10]   Habib Horry, Thomas Charrier, Marie-José Durand, Bernard Vrignaud, Pascal Picart, Philippe Daniel, Gérald Thouand, "Technological conception of an optical biosensor with a disposable card for use with bioluminescent bacteria", Sensors and Actuators B: Chemical, Volume 122, Issue 2, Pages 527-534, 26 March 2007.

[11]   Douglas R. Call, Monica K. Borucki, Frank J. Loge, "Detection of bacterial pathogens in environmental samples using DNA microarrays", Journal of Microbiological Methods, Volume 53, Issue 2, Pages 235-243, May 2003.

[12]   Ivnitski D, I Abdel-Hamid P Atanasov, E Wilkins, and S Stricker, "Application of Electrochemical Biosensors for Detection of Food Pathogenic Bacteria", Electroanalysis, 12(5), 317-325, 2000.

[13]   Mello LD and LT Kubota, "Review of the use of biosensors as analytical tools in the food and drink industries", Food Chemistry, 77(2), 237-256, 2002.

[14]   Weigl BH, RL Bardell, RC Catherine, "Lab-on-a-chip for drug development", Advanced Drug Delivery Reviews, 55, 349-377, 2003.

[15]   Eggins BR, "Chemical Sensors and Biosensors", West Sussex, England: John, Wiley & Sons, Inc. pp. 1-9, 2002.

[16]   Zhiwei Zou, Junhai Kai, Michael J. Rust, Jungyoup Han, Chong H. Ahn, "Functionalized nano interdigitated electrodes arrays on polymer with integrated microfluidic for direct bio-affinity sensing using impedimetric measurement", Sensors and Actuators A: Physical, Volume 136, Issue 2, Pages 518-526, 16 May 2007.

[17]   Madhukar Varshney, Yanbin Li, "Double interdigitated array microelectrode-based impedance biosensor for detection of viable Escherichia coli O157:H7 in growth medium", Talanta, Volume 74, Issue 4, Pages 518-525, 15 January 2008.

[18]   Madhukar Varshney, Yanbin Li, "Interdigitated array microelectrodes based impedance biosensors for detection of bacterial cells", Biosensors and Bioelectronics, Volume 24, Issue 10, Pages 2951-2960, 15 June 2009.

[19]   Junhong Min, Antje J. Baeumner, "Characterization and Optimization of Interdigitated Ultramicroelectrode Arrays as Electrochemical Biosensor Transducers", Electroanalysis, 16, No. 9, 2004.

[20]   Kai Junhi; Rust, Michael J. Han, Jungyoup; Ahn, Chong H.," Functionalized nano interdigitated electrodes arrays on polymer with integrated microfluidic for direct bio-affinity sensing using impedimetric measurement", Sensors & Actuators A: Physical, Vol. 136 Issue 2, p518-526 9p, May 2007.

[21]   Niwa O, Morita M, Tabei H. "Electrochemical behaviour of reversible redox species at interdigitated array electrodes with different geometries: consideration of redox cycling and collection efficiency", Anal Chem; 62:447-52, 1990.

[22]   Madhukar Varshney, Yanbin Li, Balaji Srinivasan, Steve Tung, "A label-free, microfluidic microfluidic and interdigitated array microelectrode-based impedance biosensor in combination with nanoparticles immunoseparation for detection of Escherichia coli O157:H7 in food samples", Sensors and Actuators B: Chemical, Volume 128, Issue 1, Pages 99-107, 12 December 2007.

[23]   Serena Laschi, Marco Mascini, "Planar electrochemical sensors for biomedical applications", Medical Engineering &

Physics, Volume 28, Issue 10, Pages 934-943, December 2006.

[24] Daniel Berdat, Ana C. Martin Rodríguez, Fernando Herrera and Martin A. M. Gijs, "Label-free detection of DNA with interdigitated micro-electrodes in a fluidic cell", Lab Chip, 8, 302, 2008.

[25] Kim JH, A Marafie, X Jia, JV Zoval, MJ Madou, "Characterization of DNA hybridization kinetics in a microfluidic microfluidic flow channel. Sensors and Actuators B: Chemical, 113(1), 281-289, 2006.

[26] Karel Stulík, Christian Amatore, Karel Holub, Vladimír Mareček, Włodzimierz Kutner, "Microelectrodes. Definitions, Characterization, and Applications", Pure Appl. Chem., Vol. 72, No. 8, pp. 1483-1492, 2000.

[27] Javier Ramón-Azcón, Enrique Valera, Ángel Rodríguez, Alejandro Barranco, Begoña Alfaro, Francisco Sanchez-Baeza, M.-Pilar Marco, "An impedimetric immunosensor based on interdigitated microelectrodes (IDµE) for the determination of atrazine residues in food samples", Biosensors and Bioelectronics, Volume 23, Issue 9, Pages 1367-1373, 15 April 2008.

[28] Zhu Q, Chai YQ, Yuan R, Wang N, Li XL, "Development of a biosensor for the detection of carcinoembryonic antigen using Faradic impedance spectroscopy", Chem Lett 2005;34:1682-3, 2005.

[29] Joseph Wang, Gustavo Rivas, Mian Jiang, and Xueji Zhang, "Electrochemically Induced Release of DNA from Gold Ultramicroelectrodes", Langmuir, 1999, 15 (19), pp 6541-6545, 1999.

[30] Ahn, C.H.; Jin-Woo Choi; Beaucage, G.; Nevin, J.H.; Jeong-Bong Lee; Puntambekar, A.; Lee, J.Y.; "Disposable smart lab on a chip for point-of-care clinical diagnostics", Proceedings of the IEEE, Volume: 92, Issue: 1, Page(s): 154-173, 2004.

[31]   Allen. J. Bard, J. A. Crayston, G. P. Kittlesen, T. Varco Shea, and M.S. Wrighton, "Digital simulation of the measured electrochemical response of reversible redox couples at microelectrode arrays: consequences arising from closely spaced ultramicroelectrodes," Anal. Chem., vol. 58, pp. 2321-2331, 1986.

[32]   Schwan HP. "Determination of biological impedances", Phys Tech Biol Res 6, 323-407, 1963.

[33]   R. Ehret, W. Baumann, M. Brischwein, A. Schwinde, K. Stegbauer, B. Wolf, "Monitoring of cellular behaviour by impedance measurements on interdigitated electrode structures", Biosensors and Bioelectronics, Volume 12, Issue 1, Pages 29-41, 1997.

[34]   Farace G, Lillie G, Hianik T, Payne P and Vadgama P, "Reagentless biosensing using electrochemical impedance spectroscopy", Bioelectrochemistry 55:1-3, 2002.

[35]   Monica Mir, Antoni Homs, Josep Samitier, "Integrated electrochemical DNA biosensors for lab-on-a-chip devices", Electrophoresis, 30, 3386-3397, 2009.

[36]   Ronald Pethig, "Dielectric and Electronic Properties of Biological Materials", John Wiley & Sons Ltd, p. 186-206, March 28, 1979.

[37]   El-Lakkani, A, "Dielectric response of some biological tissues", Bioelectromagnetics 22 (4): 272-279,Wiley-Liss 2001, May 2001.

[38]   Congjuan Li, Xiaohong Li, Xinhui Liu and Heinz-Bernhard Kraatz, "Exploiting the Interaction of Metal Ions and Peptide Nucleic Acids-DNA Duplexes for the Detection of a Single Nucleotide Mismatch by Electrochemical Impedance Spectroscopy", Anal. Chem., 2010, 82 (3), pp 1166-1169, January 7, 2010

[39]   Li D., "Electrokinetics in Microfluidic. Interface Science and technology", Vol. 2. Elsevier Academic Press, 2004.

[40] Christelle Gautiera, Charles Esnaulta, Charles Cougnona, Jean-François Pilarda, Nathalie Casseb, Benoît Chénaisb, "Hybridization-induced interfacial changes detected by non-Faradaic impedimetric measurements compared to Faradaic approach", Journal of Electroanalytical Chemistry, Volume 610, Issue 2, Pages 227-233, 1 December 2007.

[41] Radke, S.M.; Alocilja, E.C.; "Design and fabrication of a microimpedance biosensor for bacterial detection", Sensors Journal, IEEE, Volume: 4, Issue: 4, Page(s): 434 - 440, 2004.

[42] L. Yang, Y. Li. "AFM and impedance spectroscopy characterization of the immobilization of antibodies on indium-tin oxide electrode through self assembled monolayer of epoxysilane and their capture of Escherichia coli O157:H7", Biosens. Bioelectron. 20 1407-1416, 2005.

[43] Allen J. Bard, Martin Stratmann, Eliezer Gileadi, Michael Urbakh, Ernesto J. Calvo, Patrick R. Unwin, "Encyclopedia of Electrochemistry", 10 Volume Set + Index (Encyclopedia Of Electrochemistry), vol. 3.

[44] Rüdiger Memming, "Semiconductor Electrochemistry", ch4, page7, 1998.

[45] R. Memming, G. Schwandt, "Potential distribution and formation of surface states at the silicon-electrolyte interface", Surface Science, Volume 5, Issue 1, Pages 97-110, September 1966.

[46] E. A. M. F. Dahmen, "Non-faradaic methods of electrochemical analysis", Chapter 2, Electroanalysis: Theory and Applications in Aqueous and Non-Aqueous Media and in Automated Chemical Control, Techniques and Instrumentation in Analytical Chemistry, Volume 7, Pages 11-96, 1986.

[47] A.J. Bard, L.R. Faulker, "Electrochemical Methods: Fundamentals and Applications", 2nd ed., Wiley, New York, pp. 376-377, Ch. 10, 2001.

[48]   Kuo-Sheng Ma, Hong Zhou, Jim Zoval, Marc Madou, "DNA hybridization detection by label free versus impedance amplifying label with impedance spectroscopy", Sensors and Actuators B: Chemical, Volume 114, Issue 1, Pages 58-64, 30 March 2006.

[49]   Scott W. Donne and John H. Kennedy, "Electrochemical impedance spectroscopy of the alkaline manganese dioxide electrode", Journal of Applied Electrochemistry, Volume 34, Number 2 / February, 2004.

[50]   Chuanmin Ruan, Liju Yang, and Yanbin Li, "Immunobiosensor Chips for Detection of Escherichia coli O157:H7 Using Electrochemical Impedance Spectroscopy", pp 4814-4820, August 14, 2002.

[51]   Ehret, R Baumann, W; Brischwein, M, Schwind, A; Wolf, B, "on-line control of Cellular adhesion with impedance Measurements Using interdigitated electrode structures", Medical & Biological Engineering & Computing 36 (3): 365-370 May 1998.

[52]   Chantal Fournier-Wirth, Joliette Coste, "Nanotechnologies for pathogen detection: Future alternatives?" Biologicals, Volume 38, Issue 1, Pages 9-13, January 2010.

[53]   Pfleging, W.; Bohm, J.; Finke, S.; Gaganidze, E.; Hanemann, T.; Heidinger, R.; Litfin, K.; "Fabrication of functional polymeric prototypes for micro-fluidical and micro-optical applications", Lasers and Electro-Optics, 2003. CLEO/Pacific Rim 2003. The 5th Pacific Rim Conference on Volume: 2, 2003.

[54]   Satoshi Nomura, Koichi Nozaki, Satoshi Okazaki, "Fabrication and evaluation of a shielded ultramicroelectrode for submicrosecond electroanalytical chemistry", Anal. Chem., 1991, 63 (22), pp 2665-2668, 1991.

[55]   Enriq ue Valera, David Muñiz, Ángel Rodríguez, "Fabrication of flexible interdigitated μ-electrodes (FIDμEs)

for the development of a conductimetric immunosensor for atrazine detection based on antibodies labelled with gold nanoparticles", Microelectronic Engineering, Volume 87, Issue 2, Pages 167-173, February 2010.

[56] Adam E. Cohen 1, Roderick R. Kunz., "Large-area interdigitated array microelectrodes for electrochemical sensing", Sensors and Actuators B 62. 23-29, 2000.

[57] Daniel Berdat, Annick Marin, Fernando Herrera, Martin A.M. Gijs, "DNA biosensor using fluorescence microscopy and impedance spectroscopy", Sensors and Actuators B: Chemical, Volume 118, Issues 1-2, Pages 53-59, 25 October 2006.

[58] Eyal. Sabatani, Israel. Rubinstein, "Organized self-assembling monolayers on electrodes. 2. Monolayer-based ultramicroelectrodes for the study of very rapid electrode kinetics", J. Phys. Chem., 1987, 91 (27), pp 6663-6669, December 1987.

[59] Capobianco, JA Shih, WY; Yuan, QA; Adams, GP; Shih, WH, "Label-free, all-electrical, in situ human epidermal growth receptor 2 detection", Review of Scientific Instruments 79 (7), Amer Inst Physics 2008, Jul 2008.

[60] Genedetect, "In situ hybridization-the issues", http://www.genedetect.com/insitu.htm, Updated 16 January 2010.

[61] Kagan Kerman, Dilsat Ozkan, Pinar Kara, Burcu Meric, J. Justin Gooding, Mehmet Ozsoz, "Voltammetric determination of DNA hybridization using methylene blue and self-assembled alkanethiol monolayer on gold electrodes", Analytica Chimica Acta, Volume 462, Issue 1, Pages 39-47, 26 June 2002.

[62] Lebedev K, M Salvador, P Stroeve, "Convection, diffusion and reaction in a surface-based biosensor: Modeling of cooperativity and binding site competition on the surface and

in the hydrogel", Journal of Colloid and Interface Science", 296, 527-537, 2006.

[63]   Grattarola M, A Cambiaso, L Delfino, G Verreschi, D Ashworth, P Vadgama, A Maines, "Modelling and simulation of a diffusion limited glucose biosensor", Sensors and Actuators B: Chemical, 33(5), 203-207, 1996.

[64]   M. Bart, E.C.A. Stigter, H.R. Stapert, G.J. de Jong, W.P. van Bennekom, "On the response of a label-free interferon-γ immunosensor utilizing electrochemical impedance spectroscopy", Biosensors and Bioelectronics, Volume 21, Issue 1, Pages 49-59, 15 July 2005.

[65]   Su-Moon Park and Jung-Suk Yoo, "Peer Reviewed: Electrochemical Impedance Spectroscopy for Better Electrochemical Measurements", Anal. Chem., 2003, 75 (21), pp 455 A-461 A, November 1, 2003.

[66]   Byoung-Yong Chang and Su-Moon Park, "Integrated Description of Electrode/Electrolyte Interfaces Based on Equivalent Circuits and Its Verification Using Impedance Measurements", Anal. Chem., 2006, 78 (4), pp 1052-1060, December 24, 2005.

[67]   Piotr Zoltowski, "On the electrical capacitance of interfaces exhibiting constant phase element behavior", Journal of Electroanalytical Chemistry, Volume 443, Issue 1, Pages 149-154, 10 February 1998.

[68]   Wei Cai, John R. Peck, Daniel W. van der Weide, Robert J. Hamers, "Direct electrical detection of hybridization at DNA-modified silicon surfaces", Biosensors and Bioelectronics, Volume 19, Issue 9, Pages 1013-1019, 15 April 2004.

[69]   M.R. Shoar Abouzari, F. Berkemeier, G. Schmitz, D. Wilmer, "On the physical interpretation of constant phase elements", Solid State Ionics, Volume 180, Issues 14-16, Pages 922-927, 25 June 2009.

[70] Robert de Levie, "The admittance of the interface between a metal electrode and an aqueous electrolyte solution: some problems and pitfalls", Annals of Biomedical Engineering, pp. 337-347, Volume 20, Number 3, May, 1992.

[71] E. T. McAdams, A. Lackermeier, J. A. McLaughlin, D. Macken, J. Jossinet, "The linear and non-linear electrical properties of the electrode-electrolyte interface", Biosensors and Bioelectronics, Volume 10, Issues 1-2, Pages 67-74, 1995.

[72] P. H. Schimpf, G. Johnson, D. Blilie Jorgenson, D. R. Haynor, G. H. Bardy and Y. Kim, "Effects of electrode interface impedance on finite element models of transvenous defibrillation", Medical and Biological Engineering and Computing, Volume 33, Number 5 / September, 1995.

[73] G. Y. Dijksma M, Kamp B, Hoogvliet J C et al. (2000), "Formation and electrochemical characterization of self-assembled monolayers of thioctic acid on polycrystalline gold electrodes in phosphate buffer pH 7.4", Langmuir 16:3852-3857, 2000.

[74] A. Sertap Kavasoglu, Nese Kavasoglu, Sener Oktik, "Simulation for capacitance correction from Nyquist plot of complex impedance-voltage characteristics", Solid-State Electronics 52, 990-996, 2008.

[75] Stephen M. Radke, Evangelyn C. Alocilja, "A high density microelectrode array biosensor for detection of E. coli O157:H7", Biosensors and Bioelectronics, Volume 20, Issue 8, Pages 1662-1667, 15 February 2005.

[76] Champagne, D. Belanger, G. Fortier, "Electrochemical investigation of biotin-avidin interactions at a polycrystalline gold electrode", Bioelectrochemistry and Bioenergetics, Volume 22, Issue 2, Pages 159-165, October 1989.

[77] Eugenii Katz, Itamar Willner, "Probing Biomolecular Interactions at Conductive and Semiconductive Surfaces by

Impedance Spectroscopy: Routes to Impedimetric Immunosensors, DNA-Sensors, and Enzyme Biosensors Electroanalysis", Volume 15, Issue 11, Date: July 2003, Pages: 913-947.

[78]   James L. AndersonEdmond F. BowdenPeter G. Pickup, "Dynamic Electrochemistry: Methodology and Application", Anal. Chem., 1996, 68 (12), pp 379-444, June 15, 1996.

[79]   Changqing Yi, Cheuk-Wing Li, Shenglin Ji, Mengsu Yang, "Microfluidic technology for manipulation and analysis of biological cells", Analytica Chimica Acta, Volume 560, Issues 1-2, Pages 1-23, 23 February 2006.

[80]   Bilitewski U and I Rohm, "Biosensors for Process Monitoring. In: Handbook of Biosensors and Electronic noses: medicine, food and the environment", E Kress-Rogers, Ed. USA: CRC Press, Inc. pp. 435-468, 1997.

[81]   Liju Yang, Chuanmin Ruan, Yanbin Li, "Detection of viable Salmonella typhimurium by impedance measurement of electrode capacitance and medium resistance", Biosensors and Bioelectronics, Volume 19, Issue 5, Pages 495-502, 30 December 2003.

[82]   Sang Kyung Kim, Peter J. Hesketh, Changming Li, Jennifer H. Thomas, H. Brian Halsall, William R. Heineman, "Fabrication of comb interdigitated electrodes array (IDMA) for a microbead-based electrochemical assay system", Biosensors and Bioelectronics, Volume 20, Issue 4, Pages 887-894, 1 November 2004.

[83]   Meijia Wang, Lianying Wang, Gang Wang, Xiaohui Ji, Yubai Bai, Tiejin Li, Shaoyun Gong, Jinghong Li, "Application of impedance spectroscopy for monitoring colloid Au-enhanced antibody immobilization and antibody-antigen reactions", Biosensors and Bioelectronics, Volume 19, Issue 6, Pages 575-582, 15 January 2004.

[84]   Li, B.; Du, Y.; Wei, H.; Dong, S., "Reusable, label-free electrochemical aptasensor for sensitive detection of small molecules", Chem. Commun. 2007, 3780-3782, 2007.

[85]   Lasseter T L, Cai W and Hamers R J (2004), "Frequency-dependent electrical detection of protein binding events", The Analyst 128:3-8, 2004.

Chapter 5 - CMOS Microcoils and Magnetic Field Manipulation

5.1 Introduction

So far, many strategies carried out by different research groups, in order to integrate electrochemical biosensors in microfluidic cartridges and some of these include various sample pre-treatments. The purpose is to miniaturize all the steps necessary in medical diagnostics and life sciences analysis laboratory. This work aims to develop a novel biosensor integrating state-of-the-art technologies that will allow the detection and quantization of biological samples. To achieve the objective the following proprietary elements will consider. The first objective is to design an integrated circuit-based impedance system for the simultaneously reading from an array of interdigitated microelectrodes and for controlling CMOS microcoils that will be used for providing magnetic field manipulation. The second objective is to develop a low-cost disposable-type microchip that consists of an array of interdigitated microelectrodes for impedance measurements along with microcoils for the magnetic field generation. Thirdly, integration of the microelectrode chip with a simple microfluidic channel interface. Fourth objective is characterization, testing and validation of the integrated system.

Recently, widespread demand on biomedical applications the microfluidic integrated with magnetic manipulations has become more attracted and got much attention due to its great potential in this domain. Two general approaches had been studied to capture and release magnetic beads in microfluidic systems. The first approach utilizes permanent magnets [1], structures of a soft magnetic material magnetized by the external magnetic field from an electromagnet or a permanent magnet [2][3] or a combination [4]. In this category, biomedical applications were developed such as mixing, transport and separation of biomolecules [5]. Using μTAS for quantitatively analyze biomolecules is readily and fast to separate and sort magnetic particles from bulk solution efficiently [6]. A commercial magnetic cell separation system (MACS) with permanent magnets has been discussed by Miltenyi *et al*. [7]. The manipulation of magnetic beads in lab-on-a-chip systems is a rapidly growing activity, which enables the direct detection of biological entities such as cells coated with magnetic particles on chip [8]. Lab-on-a-chip (LOC) was developed for DNA detection by Smithtrup *et al*. [9] by fabricating an array of soft micro-magnetic elements to produce magnetic field gradient for magnetic particle separation. A complete separation of particles performed under external field without using hydrodynamic focusing [10]. A mathematical model for predicting the motion of both red and white blood cells under magnetic has been developed by Furlani *et. al.* [11]. The second approach utilizes microelectromagnets in various forms integrated with microfluidic channel [12]. These active magnetic separators have the advantage of local addressability but suffer from complex fabrication procedures and limited field strengths. In this category; microelectromagnets has been also used for magnetic separation. A prototype micromachined magnetic particle separator, with an excellent separation was achieved under magnetic flux density Ahn *et al*. [13]. Separators with embedded planar micro electromagnets made of spiral coils [14] and ring-shaped conductors' [15] were demonstrated. Although these magnetic separators made of micro electromagnets allow switch "ON" and "OFF" for separation compared with those made of micro magnets. Note that, the magnetic fields generated by micro electro-magnets for separation are generally weak [16].

Several approaches for microorganism manipulation have been developed based on different analytical methods, such as electrical manipulation of biological cells based on Dielectrophoresis (DEP).

Dielectrophoresis is the physical phenomenon whereby neutral particles, in response to a spatially non-uniform electrical field, experience a net force directed toward locations with increasing; called positive dielectrophoresis (pDEP) or decreasing; called negative dielectrophoresis (nDEP) field intensity according to the physical properties of particles and medium [17]. The mechanism of DEP for microorganism manipulation depend on these two forces; pDEP and nDEP, are used to precisely move cells in a microfluidic channel formed between two facing glass chips with interdigitated microelectrodes array. Despite microorganisms and cells are mostly electrically neutral. Dielectrophoresis (DEP) is well suited to their manipulation but the drawbacks of this technique making it undesirable for microorganism manipulation because the fluid flow is required to lead cells into and out of the DEP cage and electrode alignment in three dimensions is necessary, traveling waves are combined with nDEP to move cells in a microfluidic channel without fluid flow. However, it is difficult to precisely position cells, as needed by multistep experimental protocols, due to the fact that the cell speed depends on the type of cell [17]. On other hand, the DEP may damage biological cells while magnetic fields are transparent to the cells. Therefore, the magnetic manipulation method is employed to overcome all of these issues. In the magnetic method, the magnetic beads are attached to target biological cells by coating the beads with specific proteins, simply by passing on magnetic moments to biological cells. In addition, and in the light of magnetic manipulation in the conventional method where a large group of bead-bound cells are all drawn at once using magnetic fields.

A new technique has been developed and improved to trap or transfer a unique cell under a magnetic field and steering capture cells to a precise location by switching the current direction [18]. This work presented a fully integrated circuitry incorporates an array of 4x 8 microcoils array. In the light of the relation between number of turns (N) and the displacement of the cell from the center of the microcoil to the edge, choosing the size of the array be supposed to optimize and compromise; accordingly. Thanks to VLSI CMOS technology, this allows making high performance of microcoil with large number of turn (N) and small displacement (s). Each row of microcoils array connected to its own current source for independent current control. The standard theory of the electromagnetic field is relevant to this domain. The main goal from designing such microcoil is creating a single magnetic field magnitude peak at the coil center on the chip surface when an appropriate current is drawn. Each coil in the system constructed from three microcoils using metals M1, M2 and M3 that are connecting in series. As long as a unique magnetic profile is required on the surface, and to eliminate other peaks beneath the last layer of the microcoils, therefore, the three coils were connected in series, as shown in Figure 5-1. The purpose of the microcoils in the two lower metal layers are used to shape the magnetic field pattern properly to produce only one field magnitude peak at the coil center on the chip surface. On the other hand, the microcoil array should produce a magnetic force on the order of tens of pico-Newton (*pN*) on the chip surface when DC current, is applied; in milliampere (*mA*) range that is required to trap or transport cells on the chip surface within the microfluidic channel. The magnetic field profile obtained using EM field to calculate the desired magnetic force. The magnetic trapping force is given by [19]:

$$\overline{F} = \frac{V\chi}{\mu_o} . \overline{\nabla} |B|^2 \qquad (5.1)$$

Where V and χ are the volume and magnetic susceptibility of the magnetic bead, respectively, μ_0 is the magnetic permeability in vacuum, and B is the magnetic field magnitude. After the microcoil array design, the overall IC is carefully laid out to minimize stray magnetic fields from metal interconnects [20].

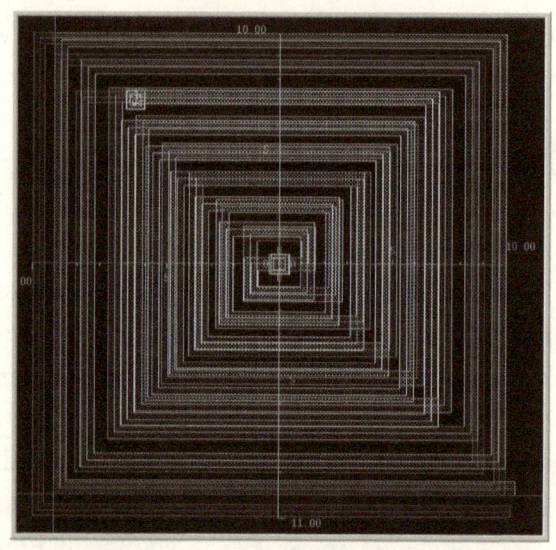

Figure 5-1   Single microcoil structure.

Microscale and even Nanoscale CMOS technology play an important role in biosensors application. Such technology allows fabricating different designs of interdigitated microelectrodes array (IDMA) and deeply differentiate itself from the conventional electrodes due to their geometrically utmost in electrochemical behavior [21]. The IDMA design offers increased sensitivity to redox cycles, improving as the electrode gap decreases [22]. Using modern techniques of photolithography and microfabrication, the sensitivity enhancing geometries of the IDMA are created with dimensions of few hundred nanometers [23]. Interdigitated microelectrodes array have the capability to improve the current response while retaining the properties of a single microelectrode, which gives them high sensitivity as detectors for flow injection analysis and liquid chromatography. In addition, sensitivity can be gained by maintaining the two interdigitated electrodes at different potentials to cause redox cycling. Therefore, interdigitated microelectrodes array present as electrochemical detector throughout the biosensors application particularly for detection of the magnetic bead-based immunoassay where both electrodes held at the same potential [24].

5.2 CMOS IC Microcoil Array Architecture

The schematic block diagram of the magnetic generator along with the control signal and current source circuits as shown in Figure 5-2 where the area of the entire circuit is 248.05 μm x 246.725 μm. The magnetic source is built using 32 microcoils in 4 x 8 arrays. Each coil, which made of three metals; M1, M2, and M3, connecting with vias, where the input current plug into metal1 (M1) and the output comes out from metal3. The integrated system described has an enormous potential to concentrate and enhance bacterial capture from samples. This integration should improve the detection limit by several orders of magnitude, shorten the analysis time and reduce non-specific detection events. The mechanism of this approach can be summarizing as a bi-directional microcoil array placed under the sensor chip; that is, interdigitated microelectrodes. The surface of the electrode of the biosensor chip relies on using recognition receptors as specific binding agent. In the proposed project, the detection process will perform through three steps process as will be unfolded in section 5.3.4. Figure 5-2 shows the layout of the CMOS IC microcoil array circuitry that performs the entire operation of detecting magnetic bead where there are two main parts, the sequential circuit that provide a DC current source, and the microcoils array with interdigitated microelectrodes array on top of it. In this system, each row microcoil connected to four PMOS transistors working sequentially as switches. Figure 5-3 shows the schematic of the control current source, where each two transistors; SW1s connected to the same clock, while the others; SW2s are connected to the inverted clock. The goal of the set of switches labeled SWs1 and SWs2 are used to change the current direction of the microcoil. Note that the rest of the microcoils rows are connected to different clock to be controlled and selected; accordingly [25]. Figure 5-4 shows the system along with the main structure of a single, identical microcoil in the array. The microcoil is built based on CMOS technology geometry and rules, where the width M1 is 0.5

µm and space is 0.45 µm, M2 width is 0.6 µm and the space is 0.5 µm, and M3 width is 0.6 µm and the space 0.6 µm, where the outer diameter of the microcoil is 20 µm. To form the microcoil the three metals; M2, M2, and M3 are connected in series with vias. The IC CMOS chip for magnetic cell manipulation is designed to generate multiple, localized magnetic field peaks on its surface by using an array of surface microcoils. Magnetic manipulation in biosensors applications is selected and preferred for two major reasons [26]:

i.   Magnetic fields are biocompatible.
ii. The magnetic fields are not subjective to the solution, which is making certain high selectivity of magnetically tagged cells.

The multiple magnetic peaks are generated to control the positions of many individual biological cells in parallel that allows more information about the testing structures simultaneously to be produced. Consequently the goal of the multiple magnetic peak whether manipulation of a single bead over many microcoils, or manipulation multiple cell over many microcoils, the bead is transported over a distance of 10 µm for each microcoil or 164 µm to leave the entire row, with the average speed will be discussed later.

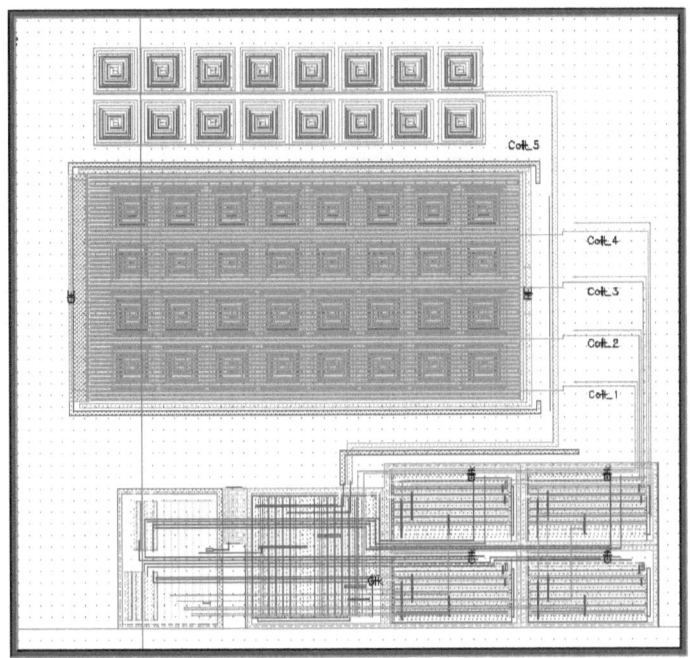

Figure 5-2   The layout of IC CMOS microcoils arrays.

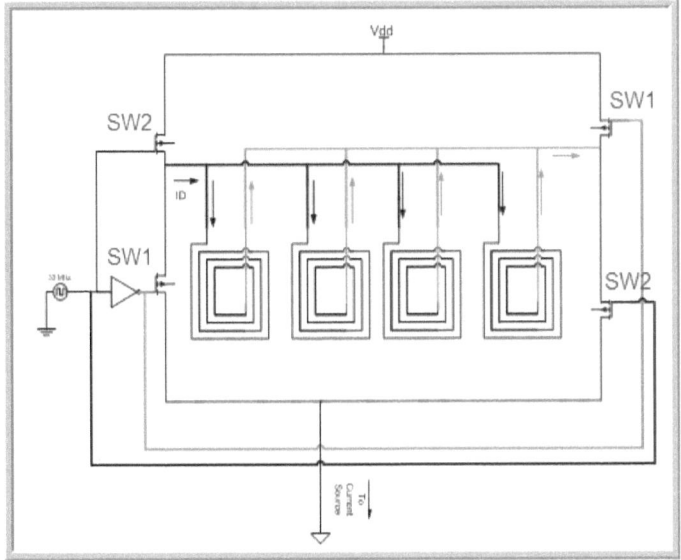

Figure 5-3   The electronic circuitry of the control current source.

The chip is fabricated in standard CMOSP35 technology (process of Taiwan Semiconductor Manufacturing Company, Taiwan). The chip is implemented using analog and digital circuits. The analog circuits consist of 4 by 8 microcoil arrays that generate magnetic field patterns for cell manipulation, and current source to provide the microcoils array with a specific DC current. The digital circuits include the control circuit to steer the direction and the magnitude of the electrical current in the selected row of the microcoil array, which will reduce the fan-in of the entire chip. The lateral size of the chip is 2.23 by 3.04 mm^2 and the supply voltage is $V_{dd} = 3.3$ V.

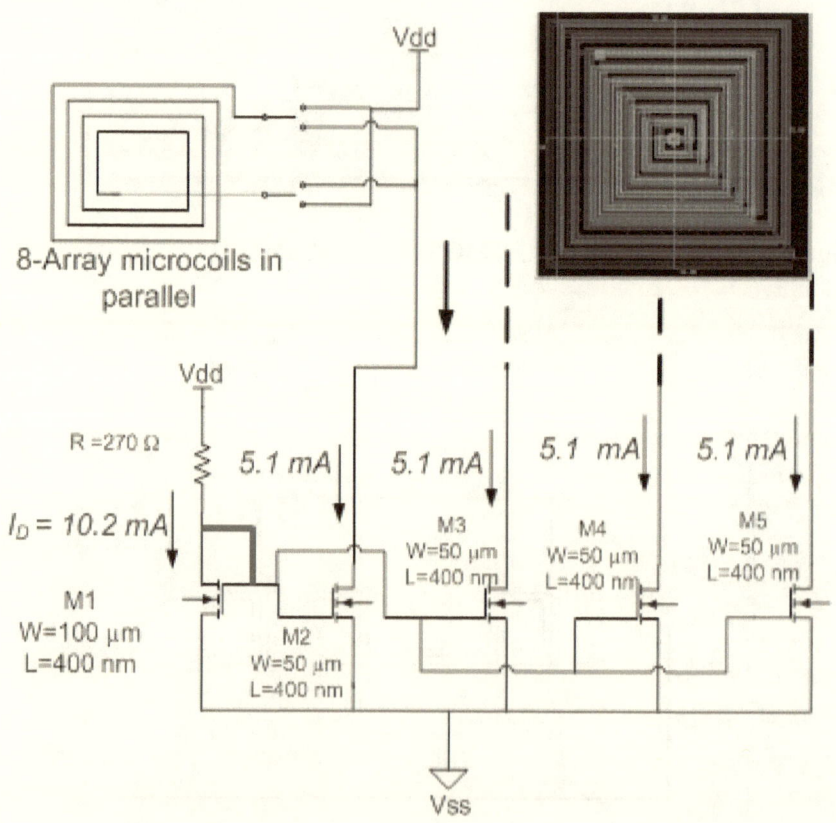

Figure 5-4   The CMOS chip with single microcoil.

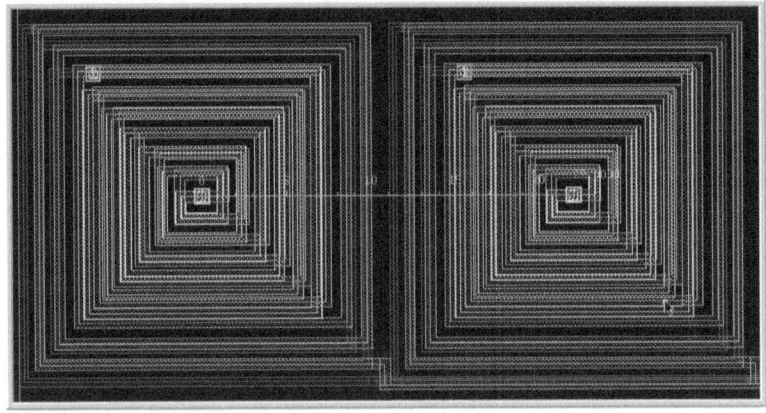

Figure 5-5   The distance between adjacent microcoils.

The chip have asymmetry array arranged in four rows and eight columns, each row has eight identical microcoils, in total there are 32 microcoils. The outer diameter of each microcoil is 20 μm and the center-to-center distance between two adjacent coils is 22 μm, and the separation distance between the edges of two adjacent microcoils is 1.05 μm, as shown in Figure 5-5. On top of the entire microcoils an interdigitated microelectrodes array with a 215.075 μm long and 114.775 μm width is placed as shown in Figure 5-6. Each finger has 0.6 μm width and space, and 188.6 μm long.

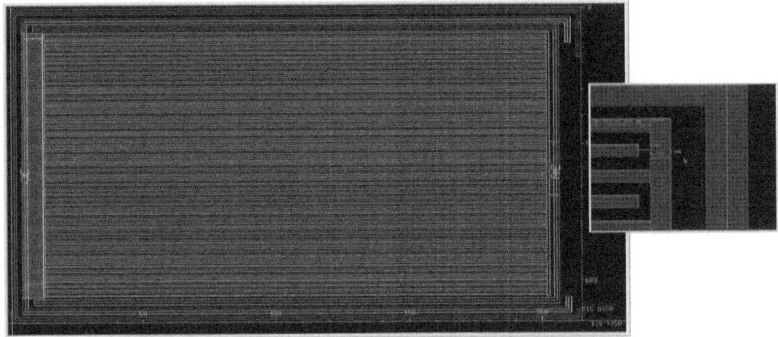

Figure 5-6   Interdigitated microelectrodes array.

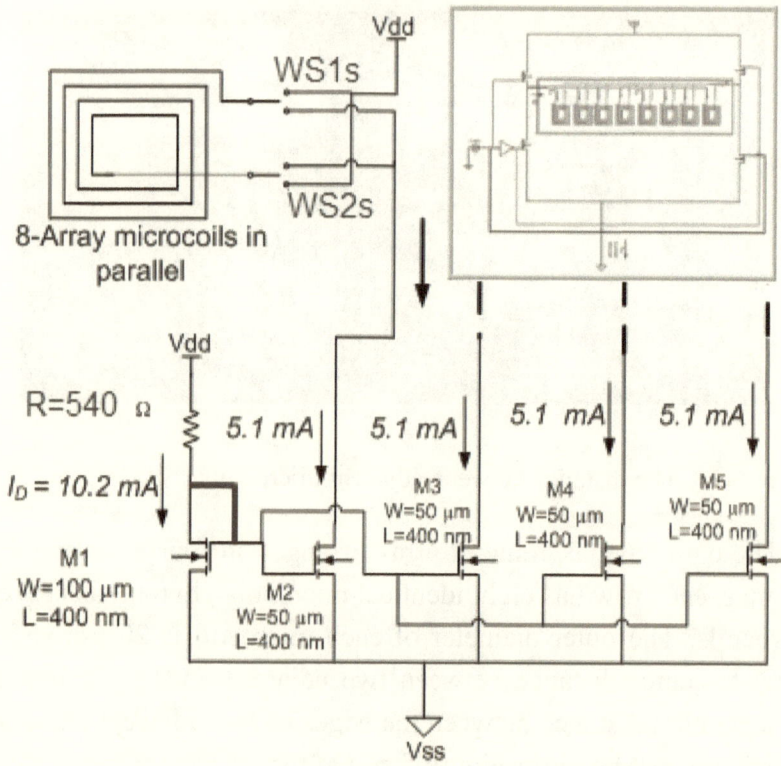

Figure 5-7   CMOS microcoil array incorporated control circuit.

Figure 5-7 CMOS microcoil array incorporates control circuit. Each row of array microcoils connected to the common current source. The inset shows the entire row of microcoil. Control circuit as shown in the inset in Figure 5-7, switches WSs1 and WSs2 are PMOS transistors while WSs3 and WSs4 are NMOS transistors controls the direction of the current. Individually activating each branch in the current mirror using a sequential clock pulse that is applied externally changes the magnitude of the current.

5.2.1   Generating magnetic field profiles from a microcoil

The microcoil designed to generate a single peak in the magnetic field magnitude at its center. The structure of a single microcoil has three planar coils, each coil is built from different metal layer; *M1*,

M2, *M3*, they are connected using vias to form a microcoil. The metal lines for M1 have the width of 0.5 μm and the separation between metal lines is 0.45 μm. The metal lines for M2 have the width of 0.6 μm, and the separation between metal lines is 0.5 μm. The metal lines for *M3* have the width of 0.6 μm, and the separation between metal lines is 0.6 μm. Strong magnetic fields can be generated with less current by having a multiple-turn planar coil in the top metal layer [27][28].

5.2.2   Design Microcoil Array

Integrated microanalytical instrument brings considerable advantages over more conventional implementations only if they provide improved performance through parallel operations, sample size reduction or integration with following processes. Magnetic Resonance Microscopy (MRM) microspectroscopy is a new field *in vivo* and the analysis of small volume biological samples that requires essentially reducing the size of the MRM radio frequency (RF) detection coils [29]. Therefore, two approaches can consider bringing such technology to the light. These approaches are solenoidal microcoils and planar microcoils. Solenoidal microcoil approach has shown potential results regarding detection efficiency and spectral resolution [30]. Nevertheless, the drawback of this approach is the more efficient zone for the detection at the center of the coil, which is not compatible with the implantable geometry for biological application. Where planar microcoils approach its detection zone is located just around the coil. Therefore, this work selects planar microcoils approach because CMOS technology can accomplish microcoil fabrication steps efficiently, and the produced transducers are biocompatible devices [31].

5.2.2.1   Spiral-Type Inductor

The storage of the magnetic field within the conductor coils is the inductor component's essential function. Because of CMOSP35 technology process limitation in the number of layers; *M1, M2, M3, M4*, it was decided to design a spiral geometry inductor. In addition, credits to spiral geometry a closed loop for the current flow in the device and a production of the linked magnetic field within the coils.

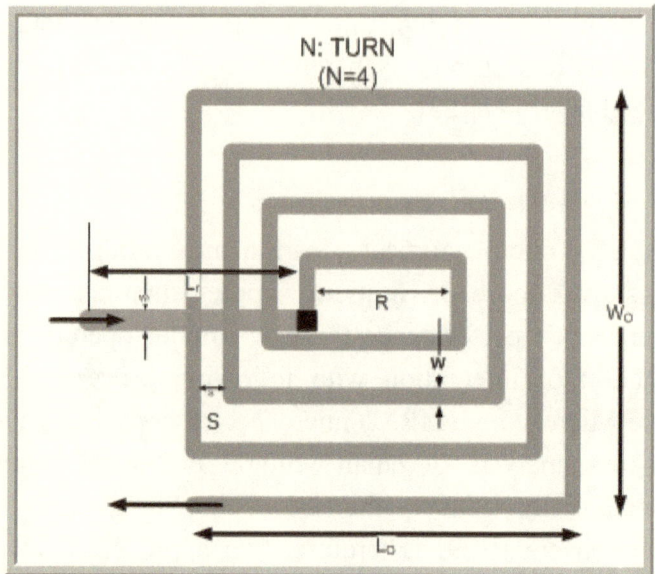

Figure 5-8   Standard CMOS Microcoil.

Figure 5-8 shows schematic drawing for the corresponding microcoil that is highlighting the parameters spiral geometry these are turn number of spiral coil (N), the metal width (W), the metal spacing (S), and the inner dimension (R) between the inner turns.

Figure 5-9 shows the layout of the spiral inductor using the three metals M1, M2, and M3 along. This configuration can hold back the metal loss in the inner turn, the unfilled coil of this configuration is illustrated in this layout. Consequently, the vortex current loss in the metal film can be diminished in this layout due to the stronger magnetic field intensity, which is observed in the inner coils.

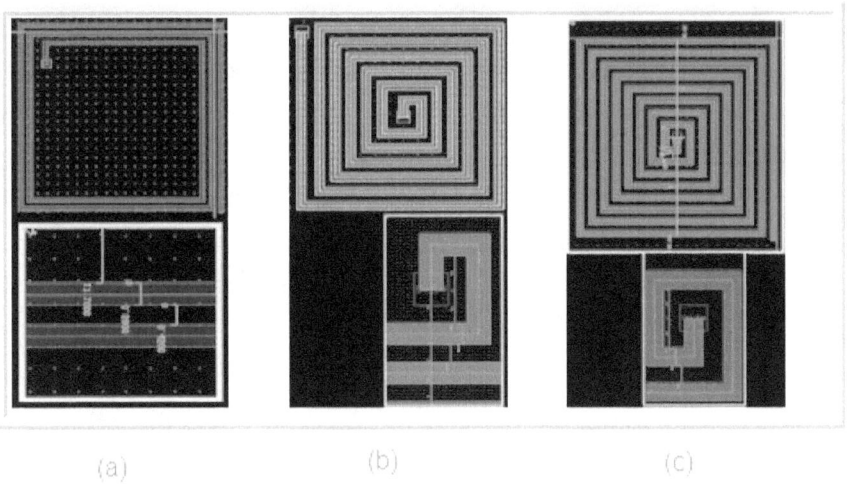

(a) (b) (c)

Figure 5-9   The layout of the three Metals (M1, M2, M3) that using in CMOPS35 technology.

Thus, there may be an effect on the linked inductance and the Q-factor value from the four parameters; N, W, S, R, that correspond to the design of spiral inductor [32]. The parameters need to obtained high-Q performance at a precise inductance must be considered by the design of CMOS inductor. The geometry parameters values for the three layers; M1, M2 and M3construct CMOS microcoil array are:

$$M1 \rightarrow R = 22.0 \ \mu m, \quad W = 0.5 \ \mu m, \quad S = 0.45 \ N = 3,$$
$$L = 10.5 \ \mu m$$
$$M2 \rightarrow R = 14.1 \ \mu m, \quad W = 0.6 \ \mu m, \quad S = 0.5 \ N = 6,$$
$$L = 7.05 \ \mu m$$
$$M3 \rightarrow R = 20.0 \ \mu m, \quad W = 0.6 \ \mu m, \quad S = 0.5 \ N = 8,$$
$$L = 10.0 \ \mu m$$

As shown in Figure 5-9 the starting radius of first coil, which is made of M1 R= 22.0 μm is larger than the targeted biomolecular sample size to keep away from field distortions due to the proximity of conductor traces to the sample [33]. The most serious reason that is making off-chip inductor impossible is electro-static discharge protection networks in CMOS technology. Regarding, bond-wire inductors have a very high quality factor, but even though they are not commonly used in voltage-controlled oscillator (VCOs) because of lack of reproducibility and mechanical stability [34]. Therefore, On-chip integrated inductors are more preferable over off-chip ones. The advantage of CMOS microcoil is not just for elimination the parasitic capacitance that produces by pad and bond wire, but credit goes to CMOS technology fabrication that shows good reproducibility.

The entire layout of CMOS microcoil arrays 4 by 8 is shown Figure 5-10 where 32 individual microcoils supported by one common current source and a unique control circuit for each row.

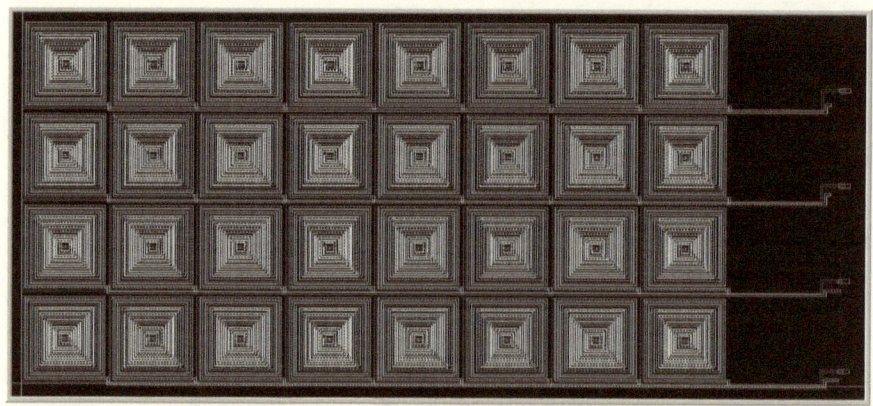

Figure 5-10 The entire layout of CMOS microcoil array using CMOSP35 technology.

Each microcoil has three coils using three CMOSP35 metals, where the first coil is made of M1 connecting in series with the second coil that is made of M2 by via, then the third one on the top made of M3 and connecting with lower in series by via as well. The spiral microcoil parameters for all of the coils are tabulated in Table 5.1.

Table 5.1   Microcoil specification and parameters

Parameter Metal	R µm	W µm	S µm	N µm	L µm
M1	22.0	0.50	0.45	3	10.5
M2	14.1	0.60	0.50	6	7.05
M3	20.0	0.60	0.50	8	10.0

CMOS technology can implement inductors in three different ways, either external off-chip inductors, packaging bond-wires as inductors, or on-chip spiral inductors [35]. The use of external resonators is not preferred with CMOS technology for several reasons. Firstly, this is due to the parasitic capacitance of the chip's pin. Secondly, the chip pin generates undesirable noise that reduces signal-to-noise ratio (SNR) performance [36]. The foremost drawback of on-chip inductors is the low-Q factor and large die area. CMOS microcoil operation, as conventional inductor, is a storage magnetic field within the conductor coils, it can be built in various geometries, and the most preferable microcoil is spiral for its larger inductance-to-area ratio. In addition, it improves the Q-factor on the expense of increasing series resistance (R_s) because of the length of the design metal. [37].

5.2.2.2   Quality factor of CMOS Microcoil

The quality factor (Q) of integrated inductors in CMOS technology go through three loss mechanisms, metal sheet resistance, capacitive and magnetic coupling to the substrate [38]. Few approaches can reduce these losses and gain high Q-factor on-chip inductors. Either by decreasing metal sheet resistance using thicker metallization [39], and lower resistivity metals [40]. The other approach by making the dielectric layer between metal layers and the substrate as thick as possible by using top metal layers, or reducing substrate losses by using high-resistivity substrate [41]. This achieved by selectively removing the underlying substrate with post-fabrication steps [42], by using patterned ground shield [43].

The quality factor (Q) of an inductor measured at a certain frequency. The Q-factor of the inductor measure how good it is, and how the parasitic are at that frequency. A Q-factor of high value refers to very low parasitic, where the low of Q-factor refers to very high parasitic. Therefore, there are two approaches to reduce parasitic, by reducing series resistance of the spiral, or by using the thickest lowest metal to make spiral inductor or a combination of both. Q-factor can be improving by making a wide metal trace but on expense of increasing parasitic capacitance [44]. The factor of this inductor can be expressed with the spiral conductor resistance of as:

$$Q = \frac{\omega L}{R} \tag{5.2}$$

The serial resistance (R) of the coil is inversely proportional to its thickness, and the length of the coil is independent on the gap that results from increasing its thickness, review appendix C for more information:

$$R = \frac{\rho}{t_{th}} \times \frac{L}{W} \tag{5.3}$$

Where; "ρ" is the metal resistivity, and t_{th} is the metal thickness. Therefore, Q-factor can be improved whether by increase the thickness or decrease the serial resistance (R_s). However, the thickness is standard and unchangeable is CMOS technology, which implies a decrease in series resistance of microcoil (R_s). As a result, the sheet resistance can be figuring out as:

$$R = R_\square \frac{L}{W} \tag{5.4}$$

Where; "$R_\square$" is the sheet resistance of the metal in Ω/square, and W/L is the aspect ratio of the device. Based on the information that was provided by TSMC through CMC for CMOSP35 technology the total sheet resistance for each microcoil; M1, M2, M3 can be determined using Eq.(5.4) for the sheet resistance M1, M2 and M3 is $R_\square = 83\ m\Omega$; 80 mΩ, 80 mΩ; respectively; provided by Taiwan Semiconductor Manufacturing Co., LTD for CMOSP35 technology. The total length M1, M2, and M3 is l= 171 μm, 278 μm, and 538 μm; respectively. The width of M1, M2, M3 is W = 0.5 μm, 0.6 μm. 0.6 μm; respectively, the calculated resistance is ended up to 28.3 Ω, 37.1 Ω and 70.4 Ω; respectively. The longest metal length is the higher coil resistance.

The variations of metal length in serial resistance versus frequency were reported by Heng-Ming [28]. As shown above, the serial resistances are influenced strongly by the dimension of metal length; the longest metal length shows larger serial resistance. The reason can be explained by the induced eddy current in metal strip especially at high frequencies. Secondly, the coil number related to serial resistance, the smallest turn coil exhibits small RF resistance this effect is explained by the less amount of storage magnetic field in this coil. The serial resistance increases as the increase of coil number due to the increase of induced eddy current in metal strips. Finally, the variations of metal spacing show the small deviation of series resistance is found by the increase of metal spacing. Consequently, the metal spacing effect plays minor role in the series resistance. In order to save the device area, the metal spacing always keeps the minimum spacing according to the definition of design rule. All of above test keys have identical DC resistance. However, the corresponding series resistance expresses quite difference in various layout configurations. Accordingly, the design of spiral coil is essential to achieve high-Q performance [45].

Variation of the metal width in each coil was proposed by Craninckx et al. [32] that the inner turn of the spiral metal line should be narrower than the outer turn, optimizing the layout and thus improve the Q-factor value was proposed by Lopez *et al* [46]. Consequently, this inductor layout, with variable metal width called as taper inductor, is a potential structure for achieving high-Q performance, by suppressing eddy current losses in the inner turns. The inductance calculation using an analytical formula is proposed to calculate the inductance for this type of inductor as reported by Heng-Ming Hsu[28]. In the light of these conclusions, and taking the advantage of CMOSP35 technology, M1 is selected to be the smallest width of the inner metal; *M1*= 0.5 μm, where the outer metal M3 is largest width; *M3* = 0.6 μm. The main microcoil structure is built from three metals as discussed above. The most contribution to the field magnitude comes from the planar coil in the top metal layer; *M3*. This planar coil has multiple turns to generate stronger magnetic fields with less current; number of turns; *M3, N* = 8. Planar coils in the second; *M2, N= 6*, and third metal; *M1, N= 3*, these layers are first and foremost used to shape a single peak in the magnetic field magnitude at the center of the microcoil on the chip surface. The three layers; *M3, M2, M1* are formed in such way to generate a single peak on the chip surface at the center of the microcoil. Therefore, in the microcoil design there are several goals had to be met [47]:

1. The final design should be conventional to the rules set by CMOS technology.
2. A single peak in the magnetic field magnitude ought to be produced at the center of a microcoil on the chip surface; this will increase the trapping accuracy.
3. The magnitude of the magnetic field is supposed to be making the most of putting forth more trapping force on the manipulation target.

In the light of these requirements, there should be a specific protocol to be followed through out laying out the microcoil structure and thus meeting the above goals; the protocols can be described in the following steps [48]:

1. The minimum width (W) of the metal line in the microcoil is determined $W = I/D$, where D is the maximum line current density (A/m) for the metal given by the chip foundry and I is the target current flowing in the metal line.

2. The outer diameter of the microcoil is similar to the size of biological cells to be manipulated, typically, tens of micrometers. This condition ensures the trapping of a single biological cell per each microcoil.

3. Once the outer diameter is set, the number of turns in the coil is swept to make sure that a single magnetic field peak is generated on the surface of the device.

4. The magnetic field patterns are then calculated using finite element simulation software, to check if it matches requirements.

5. Interconnections between the microcoil and the current sources are made using the metal layer utmost away from the chip surface to minimize stray magnetic fields.

The spiral coils are using simplified models to calculate the inductance of the closed outer core that has been developed [49]. Figure 5-11 shows a schematic diagram of the inductor model, which is to be modeled to determine its inductance value. The area of the spiral coil should be taken into account as a figure of merit through CMOS technology fabrication process. The width layer that is the spiral coil built of is directly proportional to the resistance R of the coil, where the inductance; L, is proportional to N^2; coil turns Number [50]. The parameters of the microcoil; width, thickness, and length all play an important role in the magnitude of the coil inductance and Q-factor; accordingly.

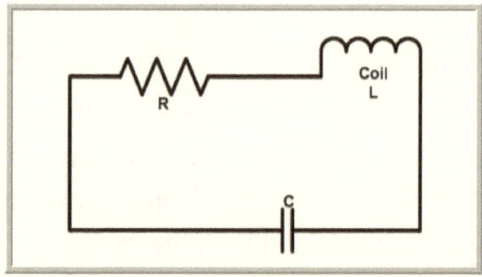

Figure 5-11 Equivalent circuit of the spiral-type inductor.

For thin-film inductors with rectangular cross sections, we proposed the simplified model for the rectangular *spiral coil* of triple layers. In order to find the inductance value we used the formulas that take the form of reluctances [51]. The reluctance R_m in the path 1 can be written as [52]:

$$R_m = \frac{1}{8\mu_0\mu_s t_m}\left\{\frac{4\left(1-\frac{c}{a}\right)}{1+\frac{c}{a}}+\frac{d}{a}\left(1+\frac{a}{c}\right)\right\} \qquad (5.5)$$

Where the magnetic permeability for Aluminum; near-direct-current case; "$\mu_0 = 1.2566650 \times 10^{-6}\ (H/m)$"; the relative permeability for Al $\mu_s = \frac{\mu}{\mu_0} = 1.000022$. μ_s is the relative magnetic permeability, t_m is the thickness of the magnetic core film. "a" is the distance between the center of the coil and the outer shunt core, and "c" is a half length of a side of the rectangular inner shunt core.

The reluctance R_{ij1} for the magnetic flux can be given as:

For $i \leq j$,

$$R_{ij1} = \frac{1}{2\mu_0\mu_s t_m}\frac{4al_i+c(a-l_i)}{(c+3l_i)(a+3l_i)}+\frac{d}{4\mu_0}\left(\frac{1}{l_i^2-c^2}+\frac{1}{a^2-l_j^2}\right) \qquad (5.6)$$

For $i > j$

$$R_{ji2} = \frac{1}{2\mu_0\mu_s t_m} \frac{4al_i + c(a - l_i)}{(c + 3l_i)(a + 3l_i)} + \frac{d}{4\mu_0}\left(\frac{1}{l_j^2 - c^2} + \frac{1}{a^2 - l_i^2}\right) \quad (5.7)$$

Where; "l_i" is the distance from the ith coil to the center of the coil, i.e. $l_i = l_i + 2(i - -1)W$, "W" is the width of the coil line and d is the distance between the upper and the lower core. The inductance in the path 1, L_m, is given as:

$$L_m = \frac{4n^2}{R_m} \quad (5.8)$$

The inductance in path 2, "L_g" can be given as:

$$L_g = 4\sum_{j=1}^{n}\left(\sum_{i=1}^{j}\frac{1}{R_{ij1}} + \sum_{i=j+1}^{n}\frac{1}{R_{ij2}}\right) \quad (5.9)$$

The internal self-inductance of the coil, L, is written as:

$$L_i = \frac{\mu_0 s}{8\pi} = s \times \frac{10^{-7}}{2} \quad (5.10)$$

Where "s": is the total length of the triple layer coil. The total inductance L of the triple layer coil with each layer of n turns can be obtained as a summation of this inductance:

$$L = L_m + L_g + L_i \quad (5.11)$$

For n = 3, 6, 8, a =11. μm, c =1.6 μm, d =75 nm, t_m=7 nm, the width of the metal M1, M2, M3 is w = 0.5, 0.6, 0.6 μm; respectively, l_i =1 μm, μs = 1.0000221, s = 0.977 mm. This generates an inductance equal to 78 pH. A full experiment has been reported by Chong H. Ahn et al [53], a remarkable notice was reached for spiral-type inductor with N = 36 in area of 6 mm^2 an inductance of approximately 20 μH was measured at 10 kHz. Usually, only n-type material is used as active region in integrated Hall devices in order to achieve a maximal voltage-related efficiency [54].

5.2.3 Digital control circuit

Figure 5-12 shows the schematic of the control circuit, which provides an independent control on the electrical current in each row of microcoil arrays. The CMOS chip has a separate and a unique electronic control circuit for each microcoil. Each control circuit is built using four PMOS transistors working sequentially as switches, where each row of the microcoils has eight microcoils; is placed on the center of the circuit as shown in Figure 5-12.

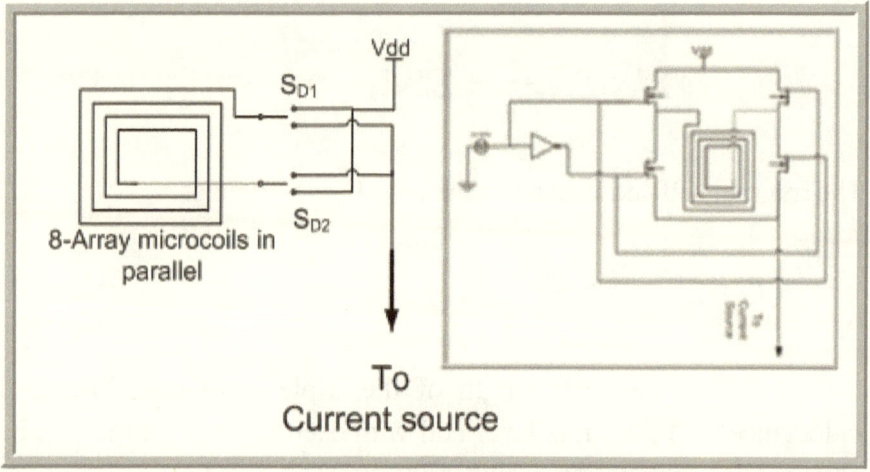

Figure 5-12 The schematic of the microcoil connecting with control circuit.

The quantity of the magnetic peaks on the surface of biosensor is proportional to the number turn of the microcoil array [55]. In a microcoil array with specific dimension (N x M) has the same current source with a current pulse. This current pulse has proportion of time during which a system is operated, it is called the duty cycle D that is defined as the ratio between the pulse duration (τ) and the period (T) of a rectangular waveform, as shown in Figure 5-13.

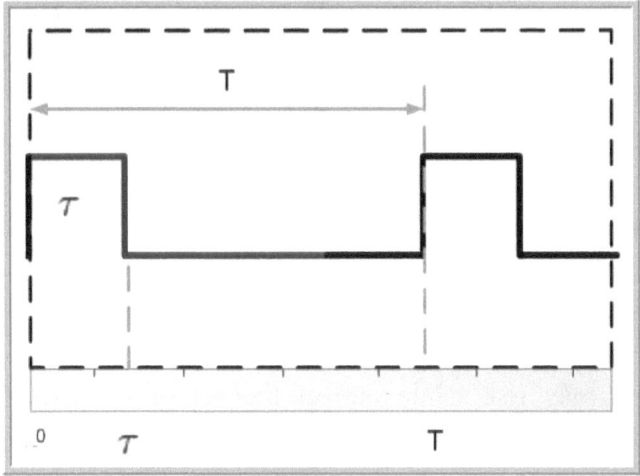

Figure 5-13 The duty cycle D is defined as the ratio between the pulse duration (τ) and the period (T) of a rectangular waveform.

In a periodic phenomenon, D is defined as the ratio of the duration of the phenomenon in a given period:

$$Duty\ cycle;\ D = \frac{\tau}{T} \tag{5.12}$$

Where τ is the duration that the function is active high, normally when the signal is greater than zero; T is the period of the function. Such pulse is sequentially applied to each row of microcoil arrays, which generates a blinking magnetic peak that scans from beginning to end of the array [56]. The importance of moving and transporting magnetic bead in submicron; in biological and biomedical applications, is making sensitivity and sampling significant in small volume; i.e. micro, nano or picolitters. Consequently, in the light of Brownian motion [57][58], that refers to the random movement of particles suspended in a fluid. The time (t_s) that the cell spends to reach the surface from the center is essential to be determined accurately to ensure that it is not released out of the microcoil, where this distance is so tiny in displacement in range of submicron. To have this concept crystal clear; the period of the current pulse (τ_p) should be less than (τ_s). Credit goes to CMOS technology speed that can handle such timing. Leakage current is a serious issue in microelectronics, a lot of work had been done to minimize its presence as much as it could be. Although, a huge work has been conducting this drawback of CMOS technology, and so far it is not entirely eliminated. Therefore, it should be kept in mind through out any application in microelectronics and particularly in biosensors applications. Consequently; a Negative Mutual Inductance (NMI) phenomena may rise while one of the set of switches (SW1s or SW2s) are OFF and the other set is ON. By definition, NMI results from coupling between two conductors having current vectors in opposite directions. In macroelectronics circuits, NMI quantity is usually so much smaller in magnitude than overall inductance that it can be neglected with little effect. In the microelectronics world, however, its neglect can result in inductance values as much as 30 percent too high where the inductance values already in range of micro or nano even picohenries [51].

Figure 5-14 shows the architecture of control circuit incorporating CMOS microcoil and displaying the connection of the eight microcoils in series at the center of the control circuit to change the direction of the current as request. The common current source is a powerful tool in IC CMOS microcoil array chip; it presents the system with many advantages. In biosensors where shrinking the sample to the nanoliter range, the volume over which the magnetic field must be uniform decreases appropriately allowing either a smaller magnet to be used, or multiple spectrums to be taken in parallel with multiple microcoils [59]. Consequently; the multiple cells manipulation; capture or release; can be performed by using this tool through creating many magnetic peaks in the same time.

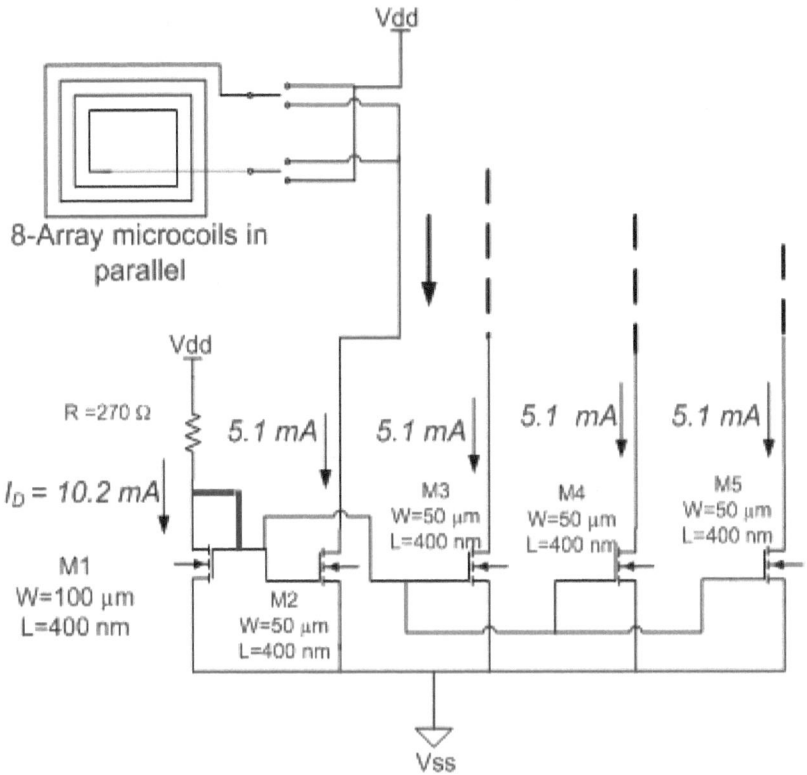

Figure 5-14 The architecture of control circuit incorporated CMOS microcoil.

Figure 5-15 shows the architecture of control circuit incorporated CMOS microcoil displaying the connecting of the eight microcoils at the center of the circuit of the control current source. Each two PMOS transistors (SW1s) connected to the same clock, while the other PMOS transistors (SW2s) connected to the inverted sequential clock pulse, with pulse width τ_{ON} and period τ_p (more details about the timing will discuss in the following section). The goal of the set of switches labeled SWs1 and SWs2 are used to change the current direction of the microcoil. The rest of the microcoils rows are connected to different clock to be controlled and selected.

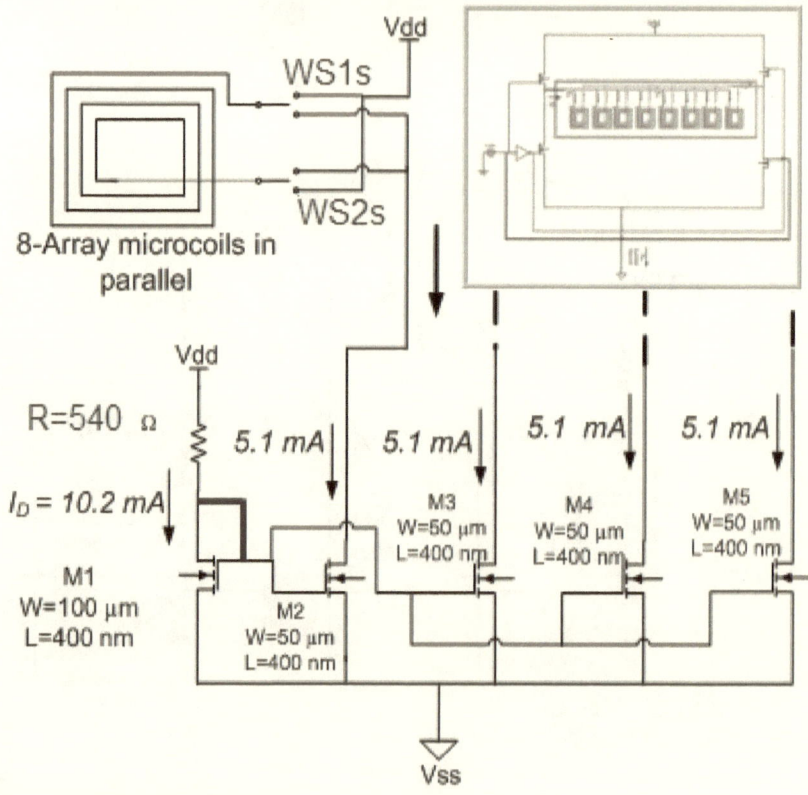

Figure 5-15 CMOS microcoil displaying the connecting of 8 microcoils in series at the center of the control circuit.

The distribution and steering of the current over the rows of the microcoils array is performed externally using sequential clock pulse for each row. Consequently; only one row of the microcoil array can be activated or more than one depend on whether the manipulation for single magnetic bead cell or multiple of magnetic cells. As a result, any row of microcoil in an array can access the current source at any given time. The current source can sink up to 10.20 *mA* and mirror to each branch of microcoil arrays by 5.10 mA distributed over the serial microcoils in the increments of 0.636 mA. However, steering the direction of the current in each row can achieve by switching the clock, or hold up the circuit by applying more positive potential to the PMOS transistors [60].

5.2.3.1 Control Circuit Mechanism

The mechanism of the control circuit that provides CMOS microcoil array with switching the direction of the current; clockwise or counterclockwise, in each row of microcoils can be demonstrated using digital electronics concepts. The control circuit built using four PMOS transistors as a core of this structure. Figure 5-16 shows the schematic of control circuit structure. As well known from microelectronics, where the threshold voltage (V_{tp}) for pMOS is negative, therefore, pMOS transistor requires negative voltage to switch ON (close).

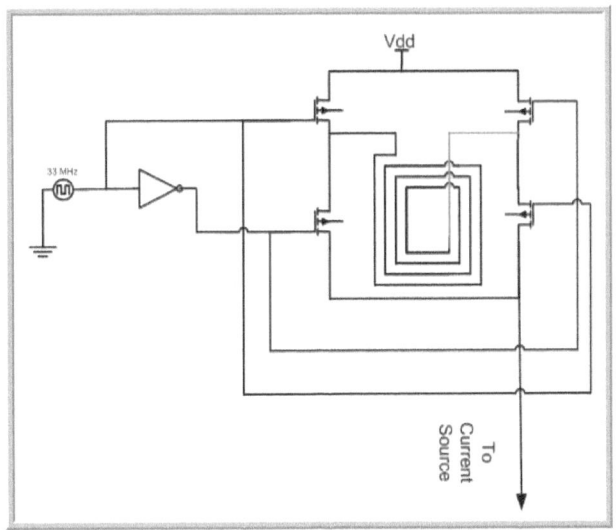

Figure 5-16 The schematic of the control circuit.

The schematic circuit in Figure 5-17a; demonstrates clearly the dynamic behavior of the circuit. When a signal pulse ($CLK = 0$) with low level (GND, VSS) applied to the gate of the two PMOS transistors (SW1s) thus the current will flow counterclockwise as shown in Figure 5-17a. In the meantime, the inputs at the other PMOS transistors (SW2s) will be inverted pulse signal ($\overline{CLK} = 1$), which make certain the set to be open circuit (switch OFF) as shown in Figure 5-17b. In case of changing the direction of the current is required to be clockwise, simply is performed by switching the inputs of the PMOS transistor SW2s to low level ($CLK = 0$) and SW1s to high level ($\overline{CLK} = 1$) thus the current will flow clockwise as shown in Figure 5-18a. Consequently, the set of the two transistors (SW1s) will turn OFF (open circuit) and SW2s will turn ON (close circuit) as shown in Figure 5-18b.

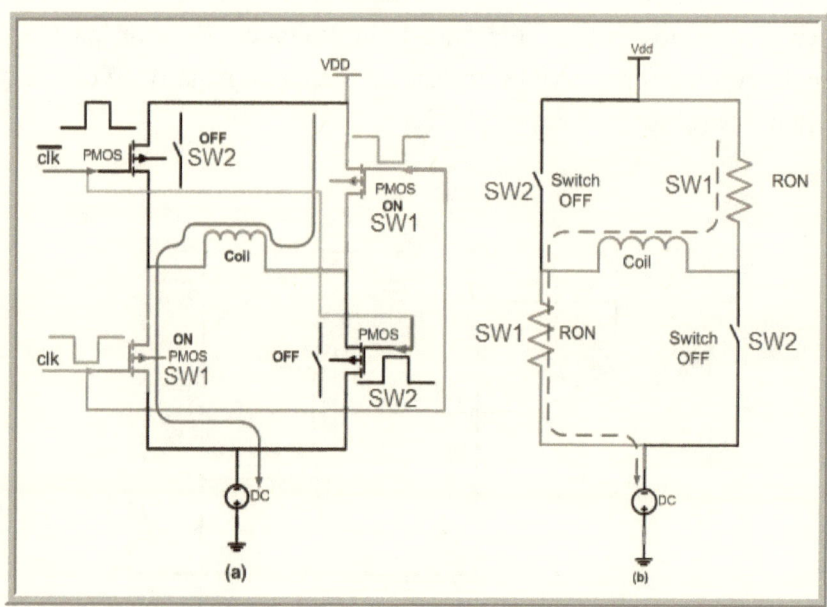

Figure 5-17 The control circuit operation to perform counterclockwise current in the microcoil, (b) The dynamic behavior of the electronics circuit when SW1s is in low level and SW2s in high level.

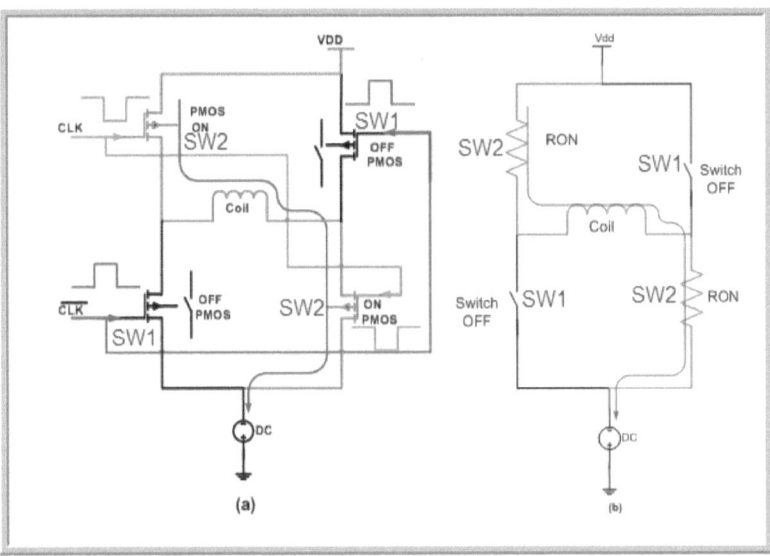

Figure 5-18 a) The control circuit operation to perform clockwise current in the microcoil, (b) The dynamic behavior of the electronics circuit when SW2s is in low level and SW1s in high level.

The objective from building the control circuit on-chip incorporated with CMOS microcoils is to provide switching of the direction of the current to perform the manipulation and steering the magnetic bead on the surface of the interdigitated microelectrode array (IDMA) in appropriate protocol. Further this technique offers more advantages in expense of cost that allows reusing the biosensor more than once in different applications, which end up to save efforts and time. The IC CMOS microcoil array incorporating with control circuit and current source, offers some advantages, particularly when the number of microcoils in an array is large. First, simplifying the interface of the chip by reducing the fan-in the microcoil is capable to be controlled. Second, it is readily to design and implement the current source because it activates a row of microcoil arrays at once. Third, the power consumption in the microcoil array is independent on the number of microcoils; thanks for CMOS technology integrates digital logic circuit to control a large microcoil array with low power consumption.

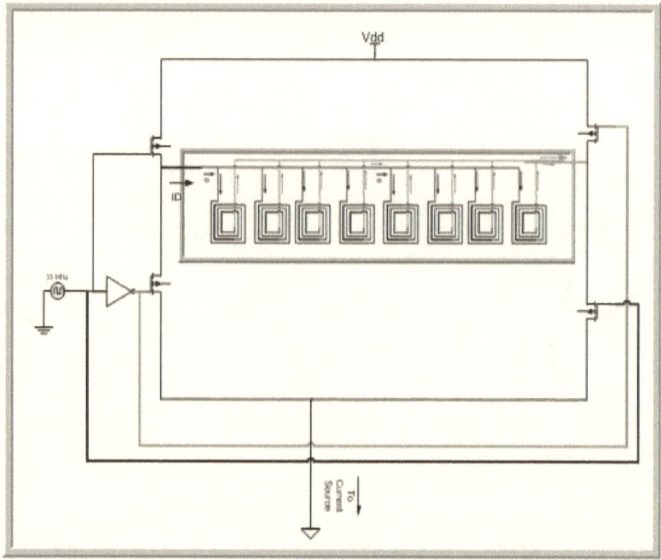

Figure 5-19 The control circuit of entire row of microcoil array.

Sharing one current source leading to minimize the power consumption and heat generated by microcoils array where only one microcoil works over the duty cycle D. Finally, the reduction in the heat generation among the cell manipulation can improve the biocompatibility of the system [61].

5.2.3.2 Current mirrors

Current mirror can be either current sinks that are made using n-channel MOSFETs, or current sources that are made using p-channel MOSFETs. The p-channel can be biased MOSFETs to form a current source. Figure 5-20 shows the basic current source analysis.

The biasing of current mirrors is readily simplified if the design performed for a specific gate-source voltage, V_{GS}. Therefore, setting V_{GS} close to the threshold voltage V_{THN}, results in very large devices, while setting V_{GS} significantly larger than the threshold voltage causes the transistor to enter the triode region too early.

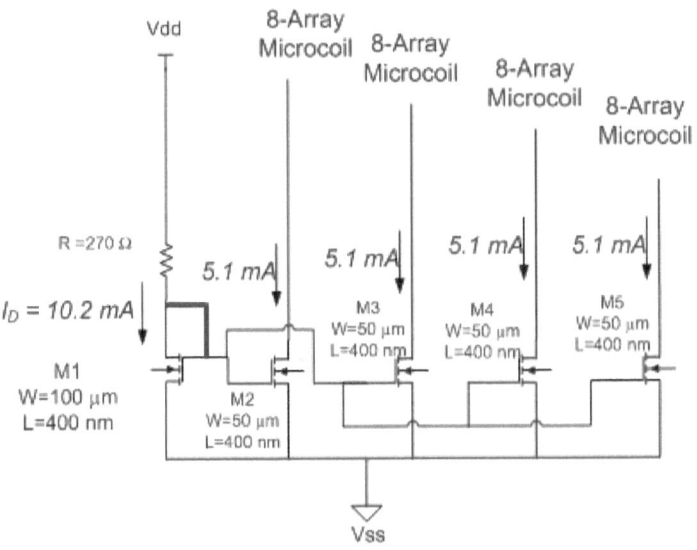

Figure 5-20 Basic Current source analysis.

In the light of what is proceeding, when designing current sources/sinks, the general design rule can be applied and set the gate-source voltage to be 1.2 V [62]. Starting the design based on these rules minimize the variables from five to two variables. Therefore, the basic current mirror design focus on the widths of the devices. The value of V_{GS} is the controller that uses to get a desired characteristic, which is the minimum voltage across the current source/sink. The drain current in the saturation region is given by the following equation that states the five variables:

$$I_D = \frac{K_n W}{L}(V_{GS} - V_{THN})^2 \tag{5.13}$$

$$K_n = \frac{\mu_n C_{OX}}{2} \tag{5.14}$$

The following table shows the most common parameters for PMOS and NMOS transistors in CMOSP35 technology, in the light of these values the analysis of current mirror is performed otherwise mention. Figure 5-21 illustrates this analysis. The current source aspect ratio is $W_n = 100$ μm, L = 0.4 μm, for $I_D = 10.02$ *mA*, V_{DD} =3.3 V, V_{SS} =-3.3 V → R =531 Ω. Design a current sink using $V_{DD} = - V_{SS} = 3.3$ V to sink a current of 10.02 *mA*. For $V_{GS} = 1.2$ V and the length of the devices as 0.4 μm.

Table 5.2   The most common CMOS parameters.

I(mA)	K_p	K_n	V_{tn}	V_{tp}	L μm	Wn μm	V_{GS}	μ_n um²/V·s	μ_p um²/V·s	C_{ox} f/μm²	t_{oxn} (nm)	t_{oxp} (nm)
2.00E-02	3.76E-05	1.13E-04	0.6	-0.8	0.35	172	1.2	4.80E+10	1.60E+10	4.70	7.50	7.70

The value of R; assuming $I_{D1} = I_{D2} = 10.02$ mA, is determined by Eq.(5.14):

$$R = \frac{V_{DD}-V_{GS}-V_{SS}}{I_D} \qquad (5.15)$$

$$R = \frac{3.3-1.2-(-3.3)}{10\ mA} = 540\ \Omega \qquad (5.16)$$

The width of both *M1* and *M2* can be solved at the same time,

$$K_n = \frac{\mu_n C_{OX}}{2} = \frac{4.80 \times 10^{10} \times 4.70 \times 10^{-15}}{2} = 113\ \frac{\mu A}{V^2}$$

$$I_D = \frac{K_n W (V_{GS} - V_{THN})^2}{L} = 10.2\ mA$$

Which gives $W_1 = W_2 = 98.3$ μm and rounded up to 100 μm. The requirement for *M2* to stay in the saturation region is called excess gate voltage, which determines as:

$$V_{DS2} \geq V_{GS2} - V_{THN} = 1.2 - 0.6 = 0.6\ V$$

As long as the drain of *M2* is approximately ~ 2.13 V or greater, *M2* will remain in the saturation region.

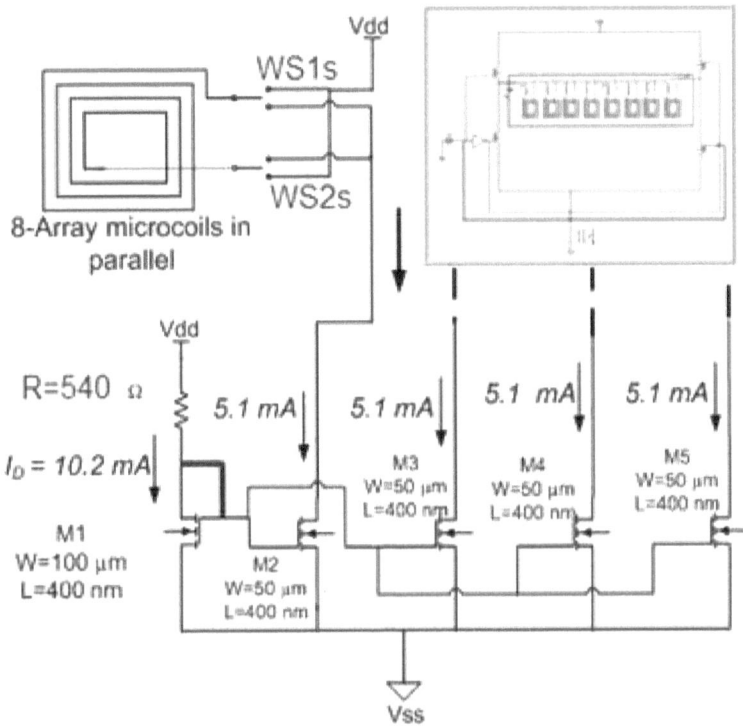

Figure 5-21 The entire IC array microcoil incorporated control circuit.

This consequence is considered particularly when the MOSFETs are biased with a V_{GS} of 1.2 V; the minimum voltage from drain to source is 0.37 V (the excess gate voltage) for operation in the saturation region. Design four equal current sinks with values 5.10 mA. Assume $V_{DD} = -V_{SS} = 3.3$ V. The design procedure is simply a matter of re-sizing the MOSFETs used for sinking current to get the current required.

The schematic of the design with new sizes is shown in Figure 5-22. The minimum voltage across any of the current sinks is 0.37 V corresponding to a minimum voltage on the drains of -2.13 V.

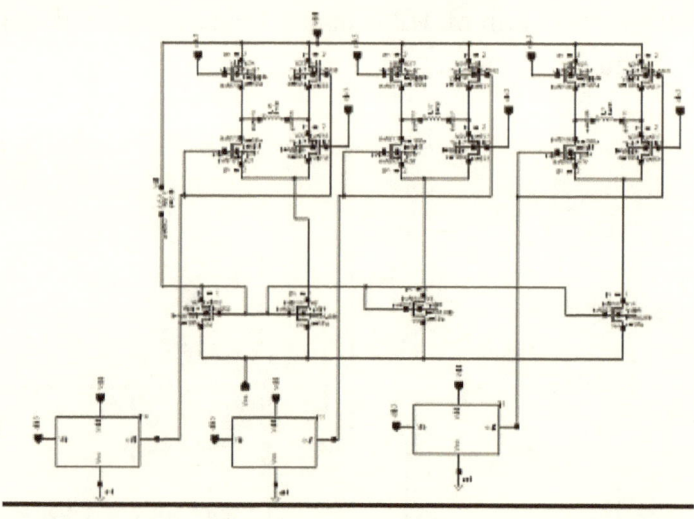

Figure 5-22 The schematic of CMOS microcoil incorporated Control circuit.

5.2.3.3 The signal-to-noise ratio

The signal to noise ratio (SNR) of microcoil transducers is proportional to the output signal and inversely proportional to the noise resulting from the resistance of the entire system and given by [63]:

$$SNR \propto \frac{S}{\sqrt{R_{coil}}} \qquad (5.17)$$

Where S is the sensitivity of the transducer, and R_{coil} is the coil's high frequency resistance. The sensitivity of the transducer can be calculated as follows:

$$S = \frac{B_1}{I} \qquad (5.18)$$

Where B_1 magnetic field magnitude produced by the microcoil holding a current. The geometrical parameters of microcoils are the main function that is capable to enhance the signal-to-noise ratio

(SNR) of the microcoil [64]. The geometry of the microcoil leads for the resistance, so the minimum of the microcoil resistance the high sensitivity of the transducer. Miniaturizing microcoil credits for increasing the performance of the transducer [65]. The SNR of the microcoil is the parameter that is limited the spatial resolution and the minimum sensing signal amplitude. SNR is defined as the ratio of the peak signal to the root mean square (RMS) of the noise voltage:

$$\text{SNR} = \frac{\text{peak signal}}{\text{RMS noise}} \qquad (5.19)$$

Improving SNR for the microcoil can be accomplished by either increasing the output signal or decreasing the noise of the transducer. Increasing the output signal can be achieved by increasing the performance of the transducer; high sensitivity or modifying the sensing surface chemically to increase the number of pathogens binding over it; or the combination of both [66]. On the other hand, decreasing the noise can achieve by reducing overall resistances of transducer [67]. In addition, the microcoil thickness is playing a role in improving the SNR and Q-factor parameter as well [68].

5.2.4   Control Circuit for Microcoil Array

Microcoil array with low power consumption requires digital logic circuit to control it, which as result provides high spatial resolution in cell manipulation. Therefore, using the capability of CMOS technology in microelectronics it can readily perform manipulation of multiple bead-bound cells [69][70].

5.2.4.1   Microcoil Array Operation

In Biosensors, usually there are a huge cells required to be handled simultaneously. Therefore, microcoil array is used to achieve this operation. Nevertheless, the drawback of this technique, which is high power dissipation associated with this operation; one cannot ignore it for two reasons; overheating is inconvenient for

CMOS components and biological cells. Therefore, a protocol should be followed to minimize it. Consequently; manipulation of multiple bead-bound cells using CMOS microcoil array technology can be easily achieved by using current source to each microcoil, which is drawn a DC current through each row of microcoils for transport or trapping of a bead-bound cell. Thanks for CMOS technology that provides high-speed microelectronics components that are capable to handle the flow of the biological cells through the microfluidic channel. Figure 5-14 shows the schematic of CMOS IC incorporated with control circuitry. The mechanism of trapping or transport a magnetic bead can be simply explain based on Brownian movement; which is the random movement of microscopic particles suspended in a liquid or gas, caused by collisions with molecules of the surrounding medium[71][72].

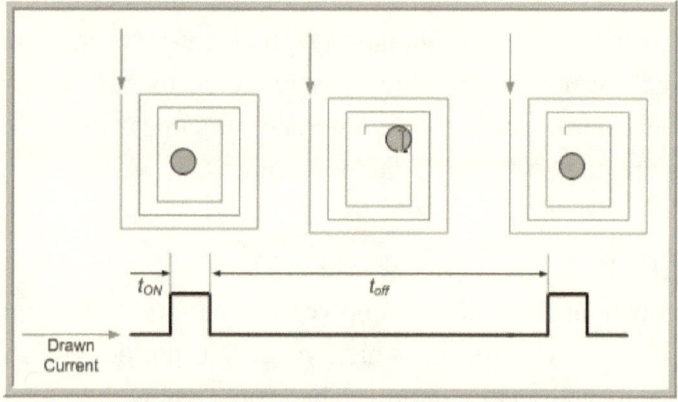

Figure 5-23 The mechanism of trapping a magnetic bead use digital circuit concept; switching ON and OFF.

Bear this in our mind; one can easily explain how to trap a magnetic bead, by applying a DC current to the microcoil array with appropriate interval (τ_{ON}, τ_{OFF}), which leads to use digital circuit concept; switching ON and OFF. Figure 5-23 illustrates clearly this process, the magnetic bead trapped at the center of the microcoil when the switch is ON; otherwise, the magnetic bead is releases and moves away in the light of Brownian theory. Thanks for CMOS speed that can capture and keep the cell in the microcoil after OFF state. Consequently, the bead is still captured in the microcoil without requiring a permanent current supply. So far, the mechanism applied on one microcoil that captured one cell, but this is insufficient through out the biosensors application. Therefore, the same mechanism applied on 4 by 8-microcoils array, where eight microcoils connected on series having the same current source, which traps eight cells simultaneously, as shown in Figure 5-24.

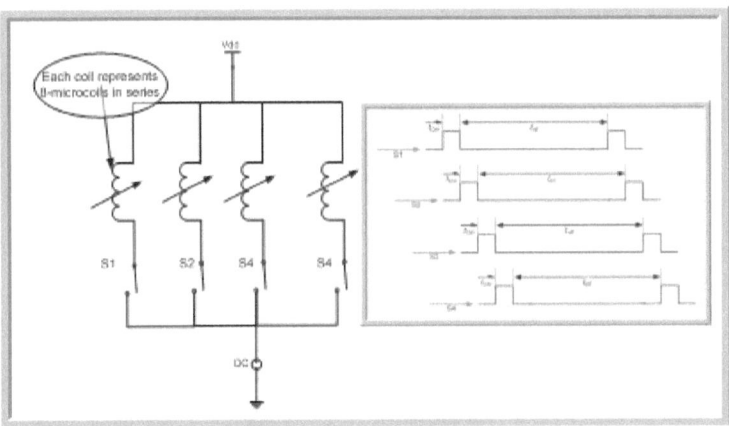

Figure 5-24 Microcoil Array Operation applied on 4 by 8 microcoil array.

While one row is ON the rest will be OFF, but still CMOS technology favor is there, so the entire trapped cells in the microcoil array remain in and never walk away.

5.3 Impedimetric Biosensors for Magnetic bead-based Immunoassay

5.3.1 System and components

Miniaturization actuators of mechanical, optical, and electronic products trend in the production spur by the significant and rapid advances of microelectronics where extensive effort has been heading for miniaturize and integrate analytical devices for Bioelectrochemistry and biomedical applications. A Microfluidic system that is dealing with micro and nanoliter of the fluid with high sensitive and throughput operation is mainly one of the outcomes of this technology. Microfluidic systems employed in different aspects of biomedical and life science, such as DNA amplifications and separations [73][74], magnetic cell sorting [75][76].

Immunoassay is bioelectrochemistry (BEC) technique where electrochemical fundamentals and techniques are employed to investigate processes of biological application that measures the concentration of a biological sample because of the specific interaction of an antibody; i.e. immunoglobulin, to antigen, where the antibodies (*Ab*) are generally used in the growth of biosensors application for their binding affinity with small molecules. BEC approach has the capability to detect the current in either case Faradaic or capacitive, in between the electrodes [77]. The magnetic bead-based immunoassay through out this work constructed from electrochemical sensor represents by IDMA on the top of CMOS microcoil array incorporated with signal-processing unit. The integrated circuit was fabricated based on CMOSP35 technology provided by CMC employing electrochemical impedance spectroscopy for magnetic bead-based immunoassay [78].

5.3.2   *Impedimetric Biosensors based on CMOS technology*

Biosensor is an analytical transducer that detects a biological response into a quantifiable and processed electrical signal. Typically; biosensor are built using bioreceptors that specifically attach to the analyte, surface architecture where a specific biological environment presents, the transducer component. As a result, the signal transformed to an electronic signal and amplified by an electronics circuit then processing to physical parameter. Biosensors applications can be conducted in biomedical, biomedicine, biological, and in life science domains. They can be to analyze environmental samples, accordingly. Biosensor research has experienced explosive growth over the last two decades. The designer of biosensors should first define the biocatalyst to control interaction between the bioreceptors and surface architecture. The second point a designer must consider is the sensor response accurate and free of noise. The third point is the size as a figure of merit in biosensor; therefore, it should be as small as the technology possibly permits. The fourth point is biosensor capability to provide real-time analysis. Finally, the above should not be on expense of the cost and complexity [79].

Fabrication the microfluidic channel and electrochemical sensor structures integrated on MLoC system is still not straightforward bringing an additional challenge to be overcome by technology in order to use this type of sensors; massively. Further, the great advantage of integrating biosensors into a MLoC system should be the reduction in sample and reagents volumes. However, to fully achieve this and bring these devices into profitable commercialization it needs to integrate the sample preparation protocol into the MLoC system.

Figure 5-25 shows the configuration of IDMA on the top of microcoil. This introduces many other challenges such as a priori smart design, simplification, and combination of the different protocol steps, or the interconnection of different blocks and its dead fluid volumes reduction. In addition, the choice of the right MLoC material for the application as well as the reduction in the final production costs are also issues and that could be great impediments to the onset of industrial and social interest.

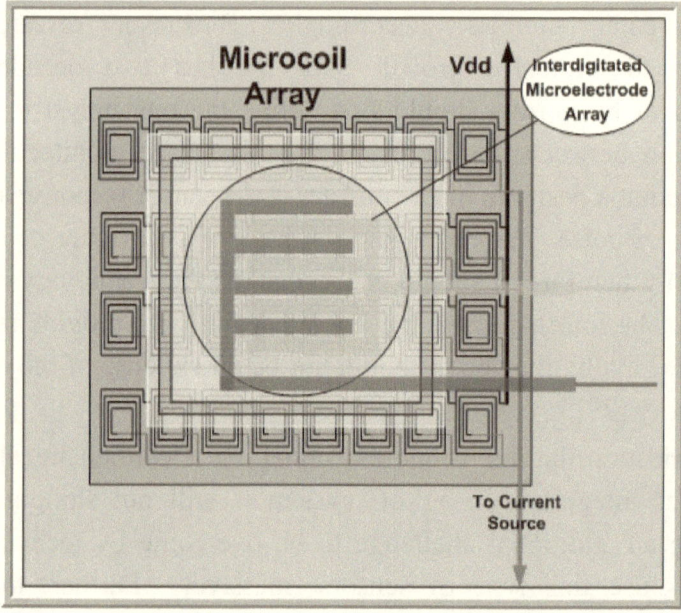

Figure 5-25 The configuration of IDMA on the top of microcoil.

In electrochemical impedance spectroscopy (EIS) the detection is based on the change of the current response before and after the target recognition reaction [80]. As long as the bioreporter sensing concentration of the biological cells presence in the microfluidic channel the impedance of electrolyte (Z) will change. The higher concentration reflects as decreasing in the impedance in turns it increases the current flows through working electrode. Such condition translates into a lower integration period leading to an increase of the output frequency and vice versa in case a lower concentration [81]. At the end, the result display by using Bode plots.

Interdigitated microelectrodes arrays (IDMA) that are fabricated using CMOS patch process provides by CMC. The IDMA had 30 electrode pairs with 197.22 μm long and 97 μm widths; each electrode has 1.0 μm of width and 0.5 μm spaces as shown in Figure 5-26. The essential step preceding the experiment running is cleaning the IDMAs with acetone, methanol, then rinsing with deionized water, finally dried with a gas of nitrogen.

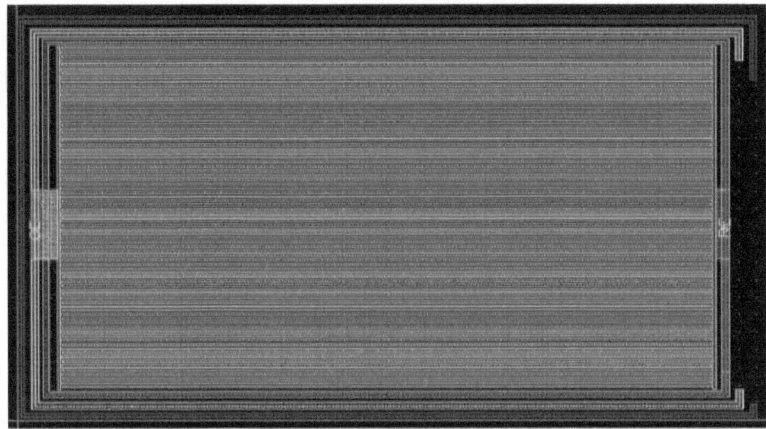

Figure 5-26 IDMA configurations.

Microelectrodes has the ability to locate down to single cell along with high single-to-noise ratio of the analytical signal making electrochemical microelectrodes technology significantly importance for single cell measurements [82][83]. To achieve CMOS chip manipulator two processes have to be accomplished, microfabrication of microfluidic channels (MFC) and then packaging. The objective of the microfluidic channels are used to move safely and keep up the biocompatible environments of the biological cells to sensing area either optical capacitive or electromagnetic. Finally, as well-known in the design and microfabrication protocols packaging is the utmost stage through out the entire procedures, which provides protection to the die from the external influence features; light, pressure, temperature, etc., and applicable, touchable, usable by the researchers. It is the interface and the connection between the microscale and macroscale [84]. The high scale of the interdigitated microelectrodes is beneficial over the conventional electrodes due to its rapid and sensitive detection electrochemical process. Subsequently, microelectrodes were scale up to reach ultramicroelectrodes to be used to measure and sense chemical reactions inside even single biological cells [85].

5.3.3 Protocols and Detection Mechanism

Planar spiral microcoils based on CMOS technology has been employed for biosensors integrated with microfluidic. Immunomagnetic (IM) technology; including magnetic resonance (MR) imaging and spectroscopy are considered as one of the most biological and biomedicine bioanalytical approaches for their advantages over the conventional techniques; electrochemical impedance spectroscopy and fluorescent biosensors.

In the present work, microelectromagnetic sensor using electrochemical impedance approach based on applied external magnetic field was exploiting for testing and validating MLoC system in appropriate conditions by detecting biological cells binding to magnetic beads. The mechanism lies on attaching of the biological cells to paramagnetic particles (PMP) at the surface of interdigitated microelectrodes due to applied magnetic field, thereafter impedimetric detection is performed to analyze and study the behavior of the biomolecular in the microfluidic channel. As aforementioned in section 2.2.2, the double layer capacitance in the electrolyte behaves alike two parallel plates' theory.

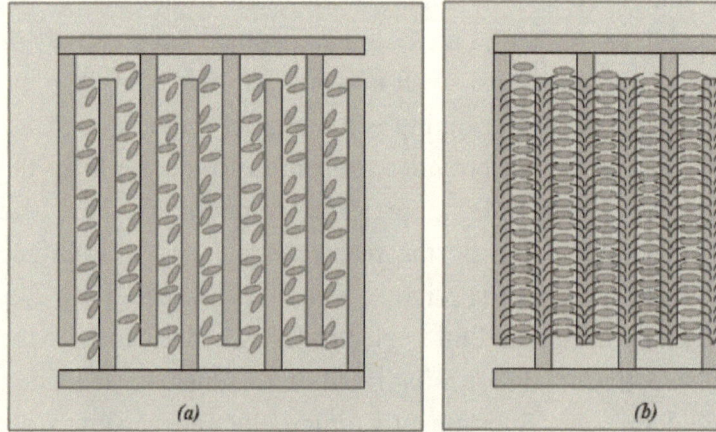

Figure 5-27 The sensing surface covered by biological cells (a) before and (b) after applying magnetic field.

For impedimetric detection biological cells, a suitable frequency should be selected under a specific magnetic field applied, in presence of biological cells, binding to the surface of the electrodes via the biomolecular recognition of antibodies along with magnetic beads therefore the entire system will be provoked and the variation will be detectable and measurable. In addition, the geometries of the electrodes and interface gap between electrolyte and electrode are playing a significant role in the cell constant. As soon as the surface of the sensing transducer modified by filling it with biomolecular sample as a new dielectric in between the interdigitated electrodes leading to variation in the impedance Z_T components; real part Z_{Re} the resistance of the solution increased and the imaginary one Z_{Im} decrease the double layer capacitance accordingly:

$$Z_T = Z_{Re} + Z_{Im} \tag{5.20}$$

$$Z_{Re} = R_{sol} \tag{5.21}$$

$$Z_{Im} = \frac{1}{j\omega C_{dl}} = \frac{-j}{\omega C_{dl}} \tag{5.22}$$

In the presence of magnetic field force, the biomolecular particles will align and dense causing the situation more different from before where the magnitude of the alteration in the cell constant significantly relies on both the size and area of the sensing surface covered by biomolecular particles, as shown in Figure 5-27. For that reason; the magnetic beads size has essential role on influence the behavior of the signal output. The largest magnetic beads utilized as label the strongest biomolecular event results the highest performance of the transducer gain. On the other hand, where the covered area is matter using small magnetic bead does not lead to the same result but worst due to the increase of active particles motion leading to loose the strength of the output signal [86]. The detection setup is illustrated in Figure 5-28. In this setup, a bi-directional microcoil array placed under the sensor chip that is, interdigitated microelectrodes.

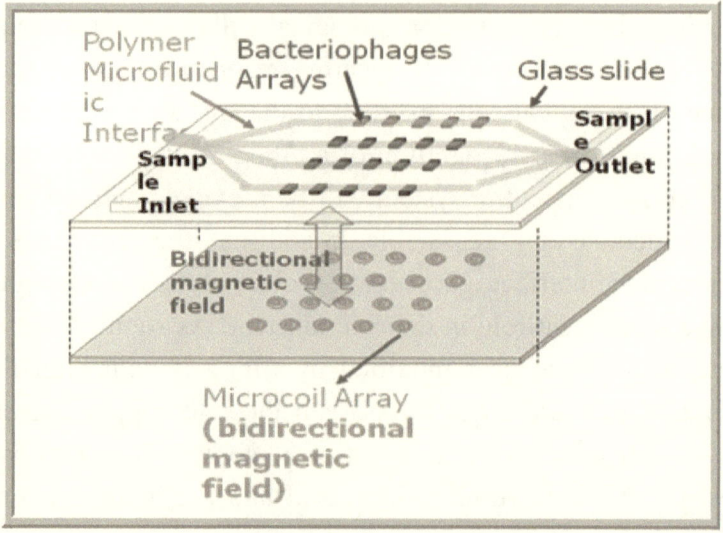

Figure 5-28 Illustration of the integrated magnetic field array setup.

The integrated system as described here will have an enormous potential to concentrate and enhance bacterial capture from samples. This integration should improve the detection limit by several orders of magnitude, shorten the analysis and reduce non-specific detection events. The electrode surfaces of the sensor chips will functionalize with the recognition receptors as specific binding agent. In this work, the detection process will be in three-protocol steps process as shown in Figure 5-29.

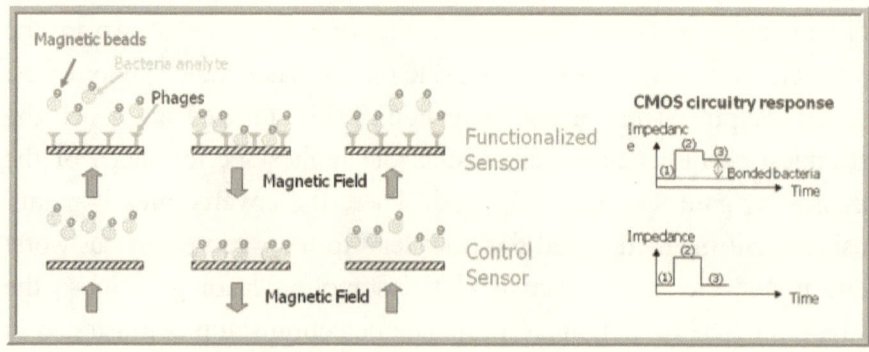

Figure 5-29 Use of a magnetic field to detect specific bacteria.

5.3.4   The CMOS Microcoil Behavior

IDMA was connected to both the control and functionalized biosensor probes, and other terminals; the reference and counter electrodes were internally connected to embed signal-processing unit. Impedance measurements have been accomplished using the build-in signal-processing unit as readout circuit; the output signal is a real-time frequency. For further studying impedance analyzer may use to get impedance versus frequency to plot bode diagram. For bacteria growth on the sensing surface an incubator made of a water-jacketed glass vial (Bioanalytical System, West Lafeyette, IN), containing a small amount of Brain Heart Infusion; (BHI Broth) that is used for the cultivation of a wide variety of microorganisms, including bacteria, yeasts and molds. The temperature of the BHI broth should be controlled and fixed at 37 °C using circulating water in the water-jacketed glass vial from a thermostatic water bath. Thereafter, the BHI broth is then vaccinating with a specific pathogen culture at a desired bacterial concentration. As soon as the aforementioned step ready then the impedance measurement proceeds right away by applying AC signal to the active layer; IDMA array, with amplitude of $\pm 5\,mV$ over a range of frequency from low to high. Afterward readings for impedance versus bacterial growth time recording to analyze the situation using Bode plot. For each run the active layer should be washing and rinsing by alcohol and deionized water; respectively.

Biosensors based electrochemical impedimetric technique besides the aforementioned advantages of IDMAs, it can be of multiple using as long neither contamination nor biorecognition element attached directly on the surface of IDMA. In addition, this technique improves the signal to noise ratio due to decrease the background noise that causes by the non-target ingredients in the biological sample [87]. The detection system approach has the following protocol that should apply for achieving the mission of this transducer successfully:

Step 1: Magnetic beads coated with the specific capturing agent and captured bacteria are introduced over the array containing the electrodes coated with the antibodies as shown in Figure 5-30.

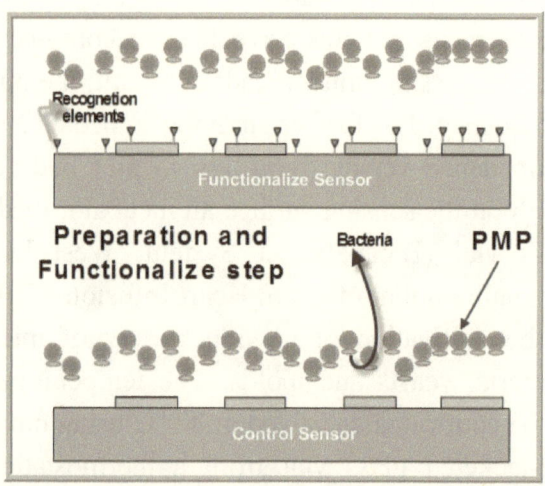

Figure 5-30 Surface sensing preparation and functionalization.

Functionalization of the surface of polysilicon interdigitated electrodes with the antibody provides specificity for the target pathogen. The figures from Figure 5-30 to Figure 5-32 show the mechanism of this technique, clearly.

Step 2: The magnet will be turned on to attract the magnetic beads, along with the captured analytes (bacteria in our case), on the sensor surface. As a result, the response of the sensor (impedance) will change due to the added bacteria captured by the fishing system, Figure 5-31 illustrate this process clearly.

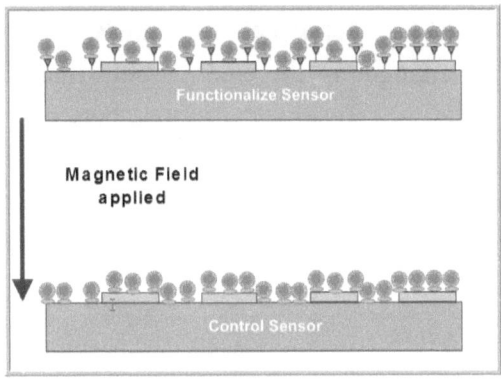

Figure 5-31 The magnetic field applied and the biomolecular attractive to the sensing surface.

Step 3: The magnetic field is then reversed, which causes the unbound magnetic beads to move away from the sensor. Since some magnetic beads are already bound to the sensor, the impedance of the sensor does not reverse to its initial state; Step 1, as opposed to the control sensor. Figure 5-32 demonstrates the detection process for the impedimetric pathogen sensor, the live bacterial cell binding to the antibody on the electrode perturbs the surface-confined electric field and the capacitance between the electrodes decreases, which can detect as the positive signal for the detection.

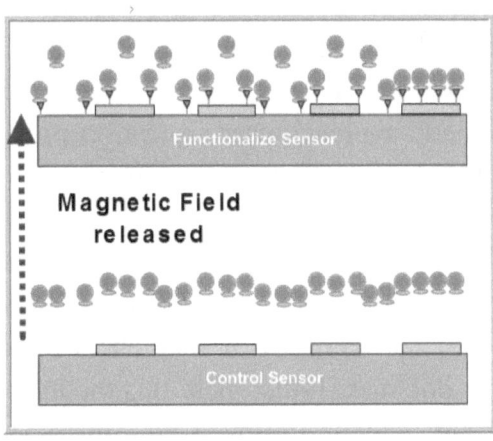

Figure 5-32 The magnetic field release or reverse.

By contrast, dead bacterial cells are not voluminous enough to induce noticeable changes in the electric field lines distribution. By measuring the difference in sensor response between step 1 and step 3, we will be able to determine the amount of magnetic beads, if any, that have bound onto the sensor surface, thus allowing the rapid detection and quantitation of the presence of the specific bacteria.

5.3.5 Magnetic Beads

Magnetic particles are superparamagnetic, when apply an external magnetic field they can instantly be magnetized otherwise released. The characteristics of the magnetic particles are micro/nano-sized spheres of iron oxide covered with a polymeric material, which allows attaching the antibody onto the particle surface where the particles size reduced to be in nano-scale, improving the possibility of handling the particles strongly susceptible to a magnetic field [88].

In biomedical, the magnetic bead is so essential, because of its size, which site in micro to nanoscale and constructing and functioning based on a magnetic field source whether it is external magnet or electromagnet. The mechanism of magnetic technique owing to the significant dissimilarity permeabilities materials, therefore it is counting one of the utmost selective approaches. The main drawback of the permanent magnet is lack of flexibility and difficulties to control it. For this reason, the electro and microelectromagnetic approach used instead to provide a selectable magnetic field by changing the current source [89]. In biosensors application, biomedical diagnostics and life sciences industries, highly demand magnetic microbeads where it is a tiny particle with an inorganic material as core, i.e. Fe_3O_4 and bounded by an outer layer of shell wall that consists of long-chain organic legends or inorganic/organic polymers [90], where this the most important part to biosensors application of magnetic microbeads. Magnetic microbead for biomedical diagnostics and life sciences industries should be standardized in size, magnetism and surface as reported by Ademtech Company. Antibodies or ligand can be attached on top of the particles to allow capturing the targets by affinity, and then the separation is accomplished merely by applying a proper magnet field. Magnetic markers for IMEA are using the capability of the magnetic microbeads by measuring dissimilarity of magnetic permeability using aforementioned transducer that consists of CMOS microcoil incorporating with control circuit and interdigitated microelectrodes arrays. Impedance measurements can detect competitively or directly the variation in magnetic permeability of the biomedical testing sample [91][92]. Because of this technique, the characteristics and the performance of these magnetic markers are rescannable and applicable because of no transducer polluted, high signal-to-noise ratio (SNR), no sample treatment, less fan-in of the final chip.

5.3.6   Magnetic Manipulation of Cells Theory

In biosensors, the behavior of the biological cell in fluids can be controlled using electromagnetic (EM) fields. EM fields construct from electrical and magnetic components. The biological cell was manipulated in different systems using both of the mechanisms; individually. The electrical approach depends on the electrical property of biological cells in the fluid that will produce electrical field to generate electrical force on the surface of the cell, which might damage the cell. The magnetic approach due to the weak magnetic fields in small size, therefore, this technique leaks the strength to control the biological cell in the fluids. Therefore, some modification requires manipulating biological cells using magnetic approach, by using artificial magnetic beads and using the combination of the two approaches; microelectromagnetic approach and magnetic approach. The characteristics of magnetic beads will unfold further details in this chapter section, such as the influence of microelectromagnets on the behavior of magnetic beads, and the manner of tagging the magnetic bead to biological cell [93].

The magnetic bead should be treating preceding attaching the biological cell to its surface, by functionalizing the magnetic bead's surface with lectins, (Concanavalin-A), antibodies, peptides [94].

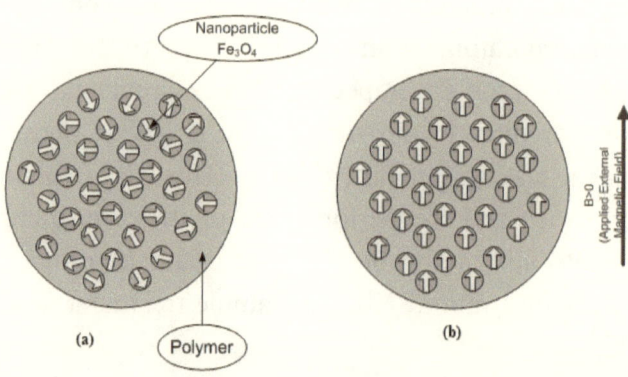

Figure 5-33 Illustrates the magnetic behavior of a magnetic bead.

The biological cells can be used by microelectromagnetic force when it is swallowed up magnetic beads or attached to each other. Therefore, functionalized the surface of the magnetic bead by modified it chemically with specific ligands will keep the biocompatibility of the microfluidic system so it can be readily bound to specific target cells. The structure of the Magnetic beads plays an important role over the manipulation process. The magnetic beads have insignificant magnetic moments, therefore the nanoparticles will accidentally leaning due to the thermal agitations as shown in Figure 5-33a. As soon as an external magnetic field is applied, the magnetite nanoparticles will be uniform and gather in one direction as shown in Figure 5-33b. As a result, the magnetic beads will expose to a force because of exchanges between the applied electromagnetic fields and the obtained magnetic moments [95]. The location of the magnetic beads right now can reconfigure by varying the magnetic field via changing the current magnitude and direction as it will be unfolded in this chapter. This property gives credit to the CMOS IC that contains an array of microcoils, which produces electromagnetic fields on the surface of the microfluidic channel. Magnetic beads are available commercially in different sizes and it is widespread on demand in biomedical and clinical applications, such as; magnetic bead with diameter 2.8 μm; (M-280, Dynal Biotech, Oslo, Norway), and magnetic bead with diameter 8.5 μm; (UMC4F-6548, Bangs Laboratories Inc., IN).

Manufacturing the magnetic beads process mainly in 3-step processes [96]:

1. Prepare porous polymer microspheres with a uniform size.
2. Modify the microspheres with a solution of iron salts.
3. Coat the microspheres with a polymer to fill the pores.

This process is non-invasive because of using the capability of the magnetic field and its biocompatibility with microfluidic system. In addition; removing the target samples that is floating in a fluid permitting quick and selective sorting of the target systems. Magnetic bead behaves as superparamagnetism because of the weakness of the permanent magnetic moment. As soon as there is magnetic field, the nanoparticles will line up uniformly and evenly along with magnetic field direction. The moment that the magnetic field absents the nanoparticles came back to its nature and randomly distributed in the microspheres. Table 5.3 shows magnetic susceptibilities of commercial magnetic beads at room temperature.

Table 5.3   Susceptibilities of most biological cells.

	M-280	M-450	UMC4F	Biological cells
Diameter (μm)	2.8	4.5	8.5	1 ~ 100
Magnetic susceptibility χ	0.17	0.24	0.18	$\sim 10^{-5}$

At a given temperature T and under an external magnetic field B, the average magnetic moment m of a magnetic bead can be expressed using the Langevin function:

$$m = nV\mu_p \left[coth\left(\frac{\mu_p B}{k_B T}\right) - \left(\frac{\mu_p B}{k_B T}\right)^{-1} \right]$$
(5.23)

Where n and μ_p are the number density and the magnetic moment of nano-particles; respectively, V is the volume of a bead, and k_B is the Boltzmann constant, μ_o is the magnetic permeability of vacuum. Typically, a magnetic bead is characterized by a volume magnetic susceptibility χ:

$$\chi = \frac{\mu_O}{V}\frac{m}{B} \cong \mu_O \frac{n\mu_p^2}{3k_B T}$$
(5.24)

The biological cells have insignificant magnetic susceptibilities compared to those of magnetic beads causing the magnetic approach biocompatible. Therefore, a significant difference can be achieved between magnetically tagged and untagged cell populations, which enable the selective manipulation of target cells. As soon as the magnetic field takes away, the response of the magnetic moments of nanoparticles will suddenly alter from thermal agitation and reach thermal equilibrium.

The net magnetic moment of a bead, disappear exponentially as:

$$m(t) = m_0 e^{\frac{-t}{\tau}}$$
(5.25)

Where, m_0 is the magnetic moment before removing the external magnetic field, t is the time fall after the field removal, and τ is the relaxation time constant for the process, which is given by the Néel-Brown model:

$$\tau = \tau_0 e^{\frac{KV_P}{k_B T}} \tag{5.26}$$

where τ_0 is a time factor of the order of 10 sec, Vp is the volume of magnetic nanoparticle, and K is the anisotropy energy constant of the particle. In the light of the above equation designing the commercial magnetic beads are typically should be matching $KVp < 25k_B T$, which gives $\tau < 10^2$ sec [97]. Having this rule through out the design, making the biological cells detach from the magnetic bead as soon the magnetic field is taken away. Figure 5-34 shows the magnetic bead when it becomes superparamagnetic when T is larger than the blocking temperature T_B. In this state; where $T > T_B$ region, therefore; $\chi \propto 1/T$ as expected in paramagnetic material. Superparamagnetic is a form of magnetism that takes place only when an external magnetic field is applied. In Figure 5-34 the temperature T_B, designate the beginning of superparamagnetic state of a magnetic bead.

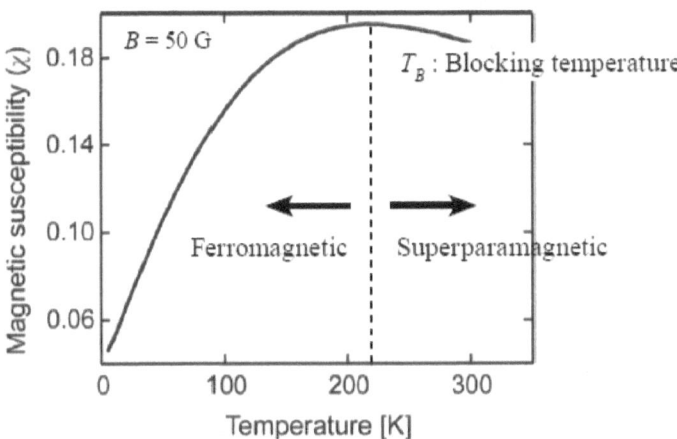

Figure 5-34 The magnetic susceptibility χ of a bead as a function of T [98].

Magnetism has lot of forms and the superparamagnetic is one of these forms; that comes into sight in small ferromagnetic; materials form permanent magnets, or ferromagnetic; materials having differing moments that are unequal and natural magnetization leftovers, nanoparticles. In small enough nanoparticles similar to magnetic bead size, the magnetization behavior is affected by temperature variations and move randomly. The time between two steps is known as Néel relaxation time (τ). In steady state; B = 0, the magnetization of the nanoparticles appears to be in average zero when the time used to measure the magnetization of the nanoparticles is much longer than the Néel relaxation time. Such state called to be in the superparamagnetic state where the nanoparticles can be magnetized if an external magnetic field is applied; likewise to a paramagnet, material except that magnetic susceptibility χ of the nanoparticles is much greater than latest. The temperature is a strong function of the susceptibility χ, it is inversely proportional to the temperature, and the paramagnetic behavior can be defined in the light of the less susceptibility χ as the temperature decreases. The magnetic beads are in ferromagnetic state as long as the temperature is less than the blocking temperature. The susceptibility χ *behaves* as monotonically increasing function of temperature, due to the thermal energy that helps magnetic field rotate to bring into line with the external magnetic fields. As soon as the temperature gets higher than the blocking temperature, consequently the thermal energy is sufficient to cause random oscillations of magnetic fields [98].

5.4   Packaging

Packaging the biosensor, which is the last step in the design, is of an important step in the entire work. As soon as the microfluidic channel (MFC) is lying down on top of the CMOS IC chip, then the integrated system is ready for operation. Figure 5-35 illustrates the packaging concept of the entire system using AutoCAD drawing.

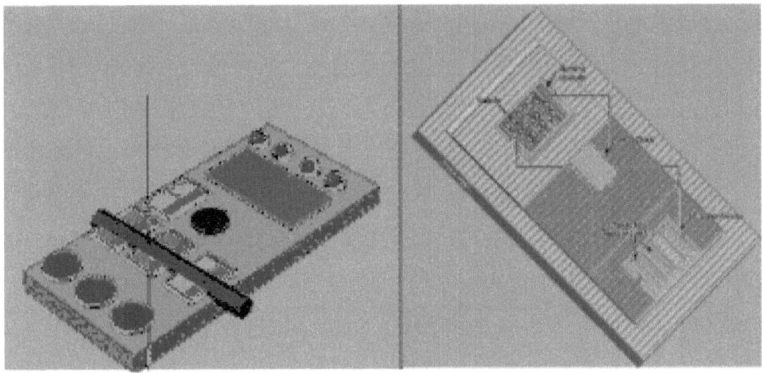

Figure 5-35 Packaging the biosensors including MFC Sample preparation.

5.5 Experiment Setup and CMOS Microcoil on MLoC System Validation

The experiment setup requires an electronic system to control the CMOS chip, a microscope to monitor the manipulation processes, a multimeter data acquisition system along with a Labview to record and analyze the output data.

Figure 5-36 shows the schematic of the experiment setup that would operate the cell manipulation system. The packaged cell manipulation system should always be in reasonable temperature.

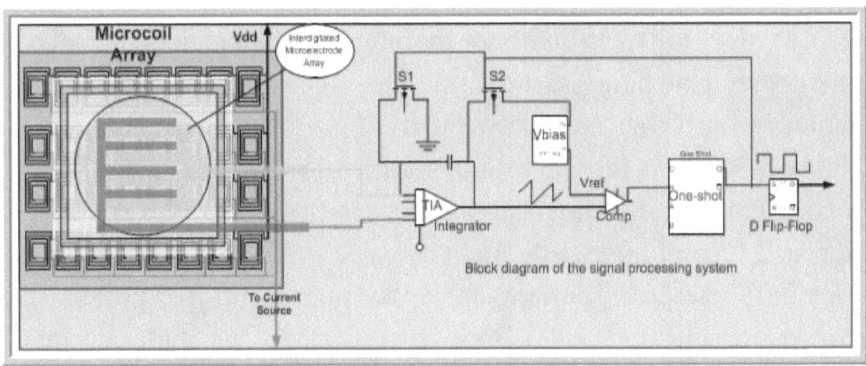

Figure 5-36 The experiment setup to operate the cell manipulation system.

To achieve the manipulation of the cell and impedance measurements using this technique, a flow control in the microchannel is required that can be accomplished using of a high precision syringe pump. Figure 5-37 shows the experimental setup for MLoC system validation. The syringe pump allows introducing the particle suspension by simple pipetting into the inlet reservoir of the microfluidic chip holder where it attached to the microfluidic channel outlet.

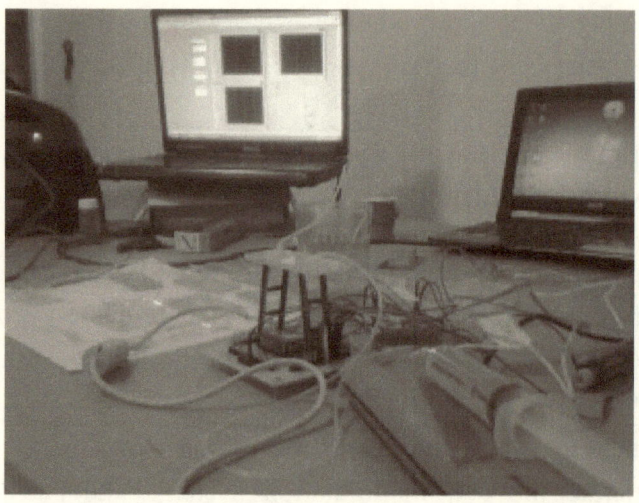

Figure 5-37 The experimental setup for MLoC system validation.

Labview software used to monitor the manipulation process. First, the matching section in the microchannel has to fill homogeneously the area between the first pair of magnetic poles. Figure 5-38 show the microfluidic channel incorporates the IDMA. Next, capture and dosing the particles can start. Finally, the course stop and a local adjustable magnetic field gradient is generated by applying externally current into the microcoil. To protect the superparamagnetic beads from any damage as their magnetic moment immediately aligns with the external field therefore the frequency that was used through out this experiment was in a range of 50-100 Hz.

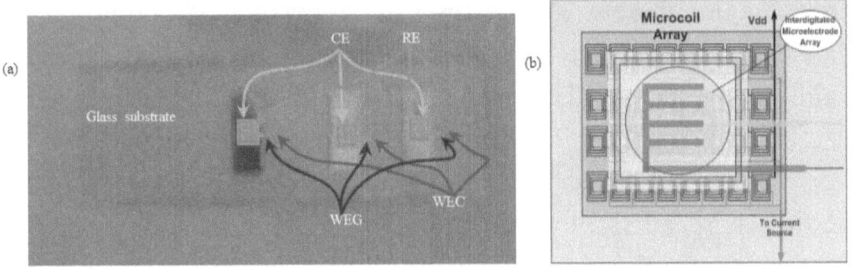

Figure 5-38 The microfluidic channel incorporates IDMA.

The external applied electrical field consents to capable demagnetization of the tips by steady damping of the signal for following release of the beads in the flow.

5.6 Labview instrumentation, acquisition, and control applications

Many applications use hook up devices to acquire data and transport it directly to computer memory. Presently, most scientists and engineers employ personal computers (PCs) for data acquisition, test and measurement, and industrial automation over GPIB, USB, Ethernet or serial ports. One time got data into PC afterward the raw data should be processing and analyzing such as biomedical data to extract the constructive information from the noise and introduce it in a form more understandable than the raw data. Laboratory Virtual Instrument Engineering Workbench; Labview is a powerful program used to simulation tool in addition to computerize testing and data congregation from an external source because of its capability to appear and operate mimic physical instruments. Such as oscilloscopes and function generators; therefore, they illustrious as virtual instruments; VI's, which incorporates with functions produces a signal afterward puts on show that signal in a graph. The basics of Labview elements are front panel, block diagram and tool palette that allows writing simple VIs to incorporate basic programming structures in Labview. The featured structures include "While Loop", "For Loop", and "Case Structure". Labview program's structure has mainly two screens. The user interface is known as the front panel that always has the 'controls' and 'indicators' required by the program to show the input and output parameters and the second is the flowchart called 'block diagram that contains the code using VIs and graphical representations of functions to control the front panel. At the end, the code allows talking with hardware such as data acquisition and on top of GPIB, and RS232 instruments [99].

Labview can take hold of hook up data acquisition devices; DAQ, to attain or produce analog and digital signals, for instance determining the frequency of an indefinite signal. In addition; it makes possible data transport over the General Purpose Interface Bus (GPIB), or through USB, Ethernet, otherwise it is capable to talk with other devices through PC's serial port. Data acquisition is merely the process of measuring a real-world signal, by fetching that information into the computer for processing, analysis, storage, or other data manipulation. The DAQ system involves PC, DAQ Hardware; in this application a National Instruments Scope (NI5124) and a National Instruments Function Generator (NI-5421) was used, software, biosensors, and signal conditioning. General Purpose Interface Bus; GPIB, is a parallel bus that many instruments use for communication that capable to bring data into a computer by using a special protocol. GPIB requires PC, Labview, GPIB board and cable. By using the different physical connections; GPIB and RS-232 Serial techniques that instruments can be physically connected to PC, afterward the last requiring step is a passport to instrument communication, which is about how to speak instruments language. This is can be provided by Virtual Instrument Software Architecture; VISA, which gives a sort of functions in Labview for transfer mutual commands to and from instruments. The way that the instrument connects to PC became is not an issue by the presence of VISA. For more information, review appendix D.

5.7 Facts and Discussions

5.7.1 Magnetic Bead Motion

Bacterial pathogens are naturally moving close to the sensing surface in micron meter range per second and seeking the convenient oxygen ambient to stay alive. As soon as a DC current applied to microcoil the combined structure of PMP and bacterium, structure binding to the surface of the active layer and captured in the microfluidic channel (MFC). Thereafter; when the DC current turned off the PMP bacterium conjugated left the surface due its characteristics as superparamagnetic but some bacterium cells may still adhere to the sensing surface. Thus afterward; to assure that the sensing surface clean and empty of cells when the experiment was done the active layer surface is treated with polysorbate 20 making the IDMA as sensing surface reusable. Surface modification chemically has credits for eliminate any remaining cells on the active layer [100]. Sensing surface making of IDMA besides their credits for amplifying the signal by recovering an electrochemically redox-reversible molecule their spacing in between fingers; 0.6 µm is smaller than the PMP size so the contact area was certainly on the surface not in between leading to keep away from potential fouling of the microelectrode [101]. The capability to manipulating PMP bacterium conjugated via microelectromagnetic is readily accomplished without any pre-preparation or/and modification in advance. However, treated PMP with a specific solution such as streptavidin will speed up the diffusion rate of the reagents into the PMP, which causes multi-layers that in the presence of the magnetic field leads to improve the sensing area then the performance of the transducer as whole [102].

Table 5.4   The magnetic bead specifications

Magnetic bead	• Radius (r_B) 4.25 μm
	• Susceptibility (χ) 0.19
Microelectromagnet	• Wire width 3 μm
	• Wire thickness 0.3 μm
	• Wire pitch (d) 10 μm
	• Insulator thickness 1 μm
Environment	Temperature 25°C =300 °K
	Fluid viscosity (η) 1.0×10^{-3} N·sec/m^2

Magnetic beads can be captured or released depend on the external applied magnetic field. The influence of the magnetic fields on the behavior of the magnetic bead in a fluid will be investigating. The Magnetic Bead Motion can be determined in the light of Brownian motion using the data as shown in Table 5.4. The switching time interval (τ_{ON}, τ_{OFF}) that requires to keep the magnetic bead captured within the center of the microcoil array, where the cell moved under the Brownian motion away from the center through OFF state by the mean displacement (s):

$$s = (D \cdot \tau_{OFF})^{1/2} = [D \cdot (N^2 - 1) \cdot \tau_{ON}]^{1/2} \qquad (5.27)$$

The diffusion constant (D) for a magnetic bead of radius r_B in a fluid with viscosity η (1.0×10^{-3} N·sec/m^2) can be determined based on Brownian Motion as:

$$D = \frac{k_B T}{6\pi\eta r_B} \qquad (5.28)$$

Where k_B is the Boltzmann constant ($1.3806514 \times 10^{-23}$ JK^{-1}) and T is the absolute temperature (300 °K).

Keeping the magnetic bead within the center of the microcoil demands strongly the displacement (s) to be always smaller than the radius r of the microcoil. Having this condition into account, means the magnetic cell will hang on to the center of the microcoil during ON State. As a result, the ON state timing can be determined as

$$\tau_{ON} < \frac{r^2}{[D \cdot (N^2 - 1)]} \tag{5.29}$$

The entire time for switching (ON & OFF states) can be also evaluating as follows:

$$\tau_p < \frac{r^2 N^2}{[D \cdot (N^2 - 1)]} \tag{5.30}$$

CMOS technology still play very important role in this field, where the number of turns is essential but apparently it inversely proportional to ON state, so to come over this problem using high scale of CMOS technology can easily produce microcoil array with small radius and large number of turns simultaneously. Having this concept into account, and taking the condition as shown in Table 5.4 and taking different radius of microcoils for the same number of microcoil turns the result in Figure 5-39 shows a remarkable notice that confirms the necessary of CMOS technology as mention before. The results is illustrated that ON timing is the smallest for the large number of turns (10 by 10) but as long as the radius increases the timing for the entire period (τ_p) and even the ON state time increases. For radius changing from 0 (center of microcoil) up to 10 µm; the period τ_p changes from 0 up to < 230 sec and ON state timing from 0 up to < 2.3 sec.

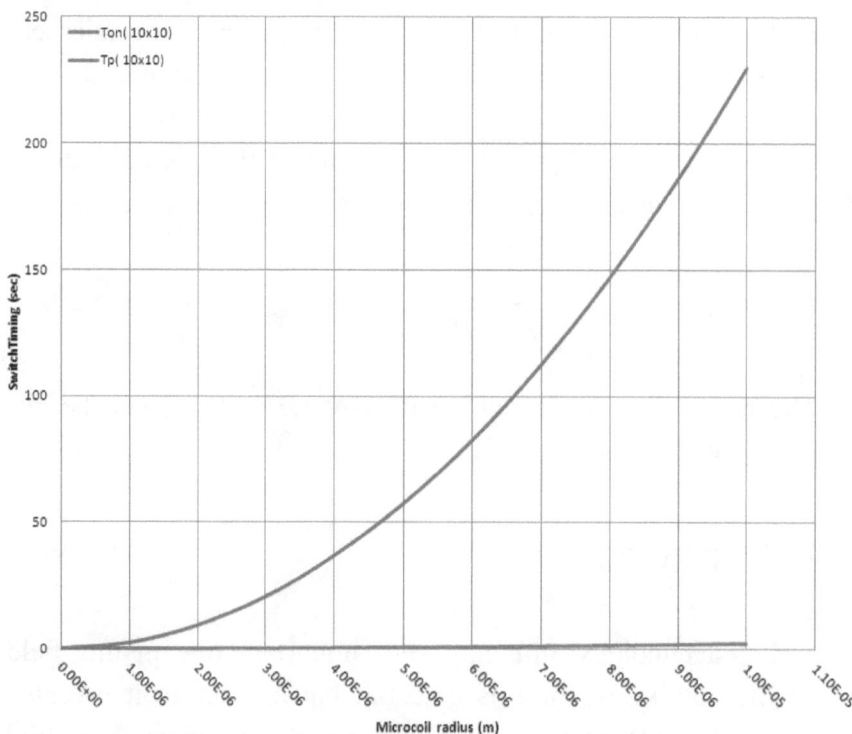

Figure 5-39 The entire time for switching τ_p and τ_{ON} on behalf of the 10 x 10 microcoil for different radius.

Figure 5-40 shows the result of a sort of microcoils having the same conditions but different turn numbers (N by N); 10 by 10, 8 by 8, 4 by 8, and, 4 by 4.

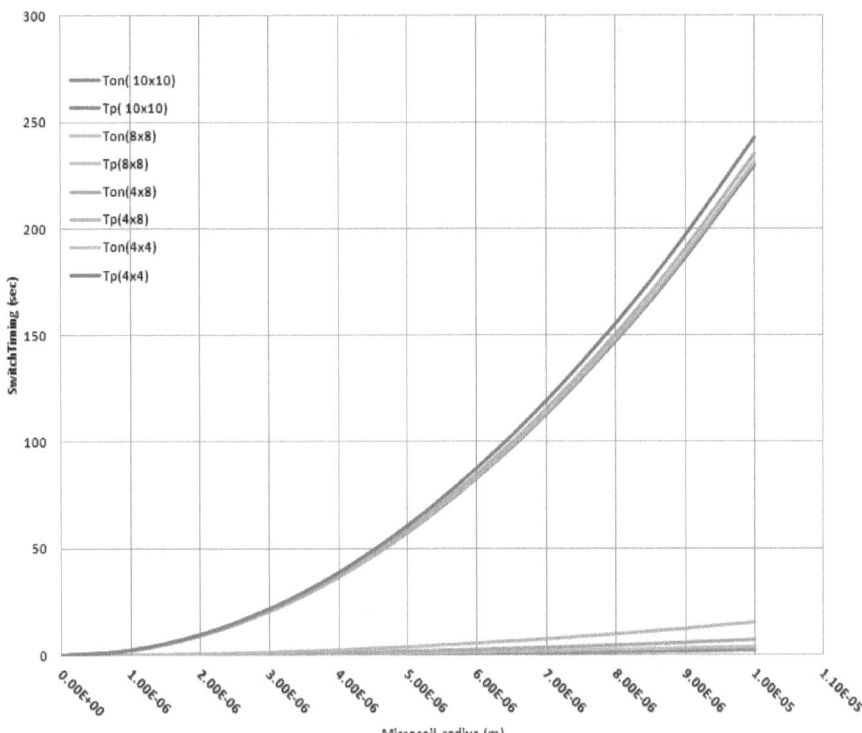

Figure 5-40 The variation of switch timing (ON and OFF states) for different radius of microcoils, and Number of microcoil turns.

Figure 5-40 shows the result for different microcoils array and the less number of turns the more time required, where the radius range for all of them is the same from origin (center of microcoil) up to 10 μm.

These conditions are easily satisfied as electronic circuits in the chip operate at much higher speed. To compare the timing required the microcoils should sort in different categories and then display the results as a histogram for easily elaborating and studying.

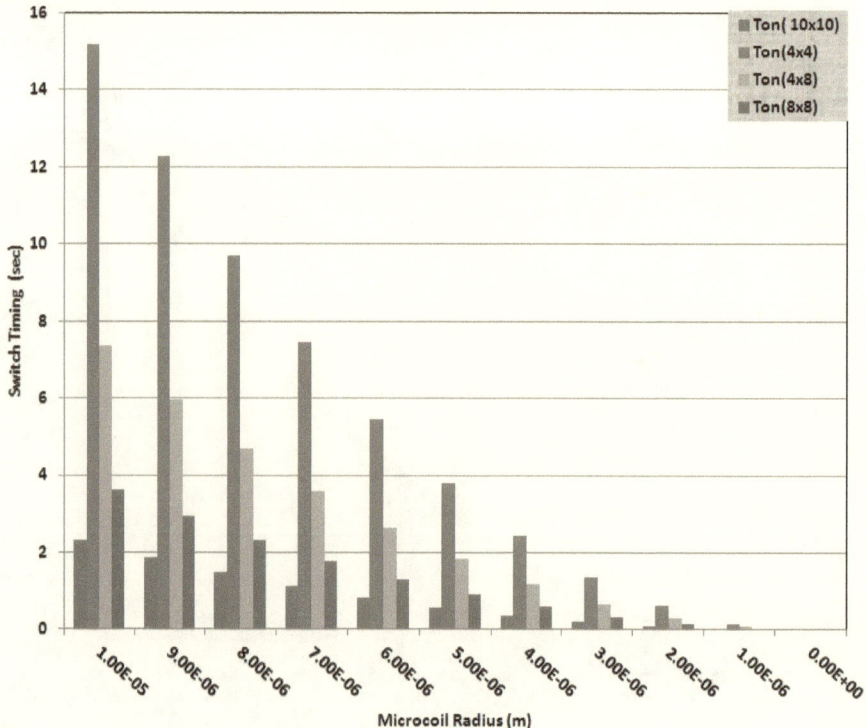

Figure 5-41 The time required for ON state (τ_{ON}).

Figure 5-41 shows the clustered column for illustrating the behavior of sort of microcoils in different number of turn over a range of radius represent the motion of the cell from the center of the microcoil up to the surface through ON state.

Figure 5-42 shows the clustered column for illustrating the behavior of sort of microcoils in different number of turn over a range of radius represent the motion of the cell from the center of the microcoil up to the surface over the entire period (τ_p); i.e. ON & OFF states.

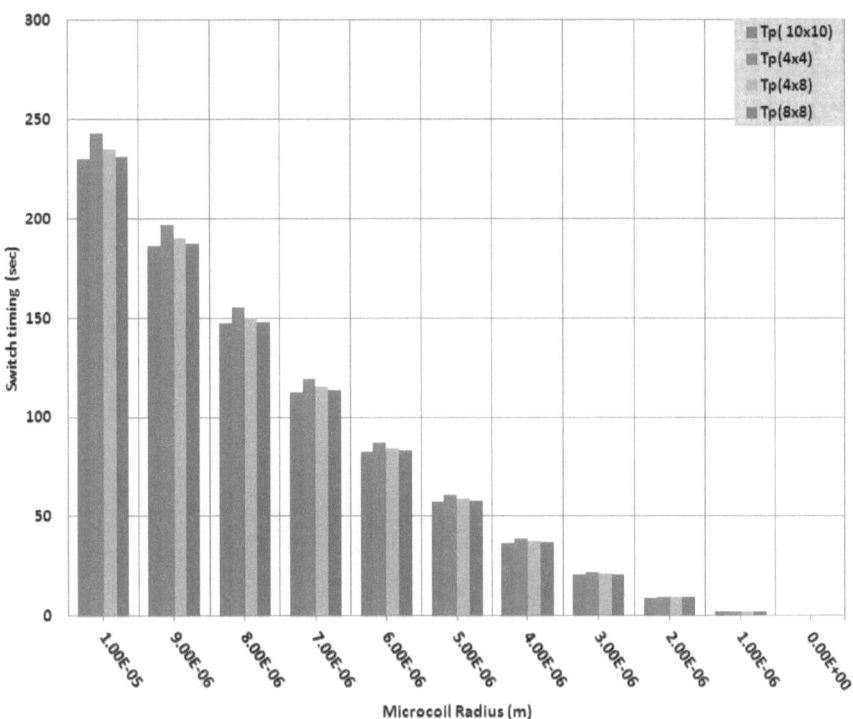

Figure 5-42 The entire time require for ON and OFF state (τ_p).

Figure 5-43 shows the speed of the cell under magnetic field from the center of the microcoil to the surface, through ON state. Figure 5-44 shows the behavior of the magnetic bead among the transport time, entire period (τ_p). The preceding sketching clearly makes obvious the advantage of the CMOS technology process to capture multiple bead-bound cells; all at once. In the light of low-power operation, moving multiple bead-bound cells in real-time it comes at the cost of an increased transport time.

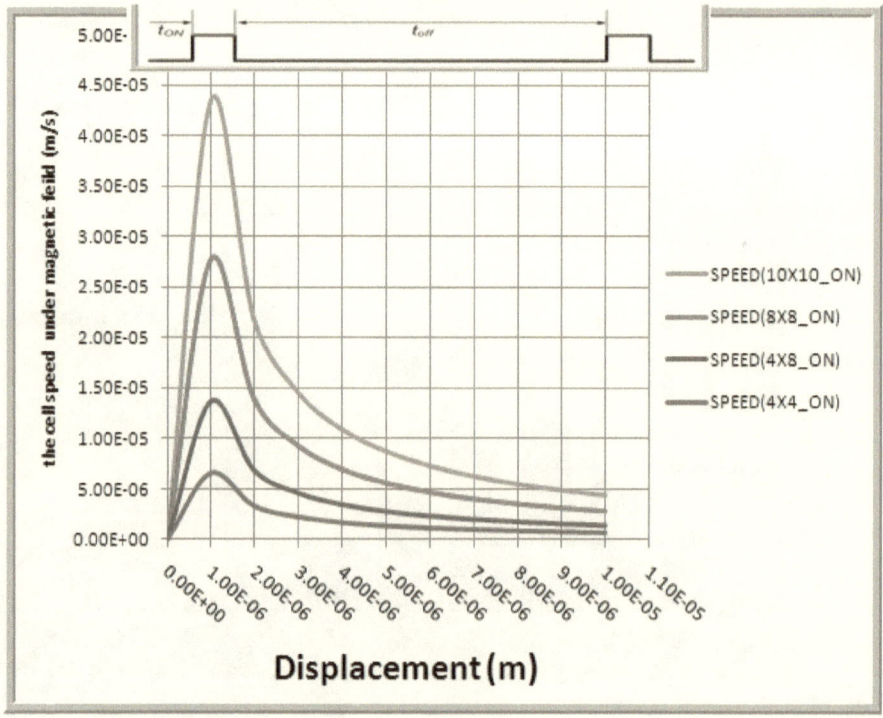

Figure 5-43 The speed of the cell under the magnetic field over the displacement (s) and the entire time interval (ON) from the center of the microcoil to the end.

This is because bead-bound cells are pulled by the microcoil not continuously but for a short duration t_{on} over the entire period τ_p. Cutback the power at the cost of the increased transport time is utmost wanted to keep away from thermal IC malfunction and to preserve biocompatible environment; accordingly.

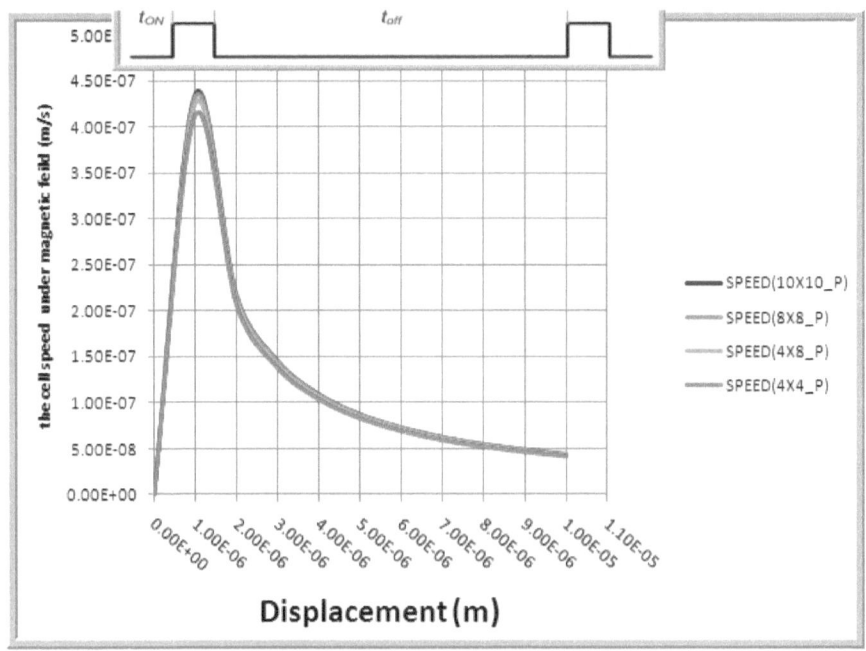

Figure 5-44 The cell speed over the period ON & OFF states.

5.7.2 *Magnetic Field Controlling*

Current source incorporated in microcoil array is a powerful tool in biosensors and magnetic bead domain. The current source can steer the entire operation, therefore; as it can be readily creating a single magnetic peak at each row microcoil; assorted magnetic field patterns can be generated by changing current distributions in a microcoil array; as well. The mechanism of controlling the peak of the magnetic field, which can be produced at the centers of microcoils, which leads to increase the spatial resolution of cell trapping; it can be achieving by adjusting in cooperation the magnitude and the direction of currents. Where during the peak movements, the magnitude of the peak remains nearly constant, but the direction of the magnetic field is changing as long as the current direction changing. Figure 5-45 shows the circuitry that performs the controlling on the magnitude and the direction of currents in the microcoil array.

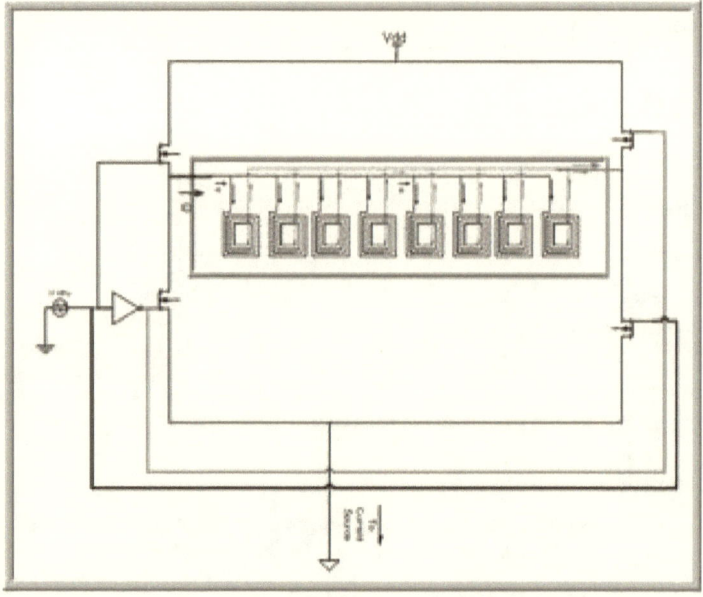

Figure 5-45   Circuitry that steers the magnitude and the direction of currents.

5.7.3   EIS technique Validation on MLoC System

EIS technique is employing for impedance measurements. The output from the signal-processing unit ended up to that the higher concentration of biological cells binding to the electrode surface the lower impedance the more current flow through CE the higher frequency occurred at the output of the signal-processing unit. MLoC system tested and validated as impedance analyzer among three conditions, one as control and the other two as sensing transducers for comparing the variation of the impedance before and after applying the magnetic field (B) as demonstrated in schematic Figure 5-27. The four electrodes configuration used as a sensing layers for the three cases as shown in Figure 5-30, where IDMA acts as working electrodes, i.e. WEC and WEG. A solution made of LB media with a specific concentration of biological cells mixed with magnetic beads (PMP). The reference (RE) and counter electrodes (CE) plug into the chip, where the output data obtained then analyzed appropriately using Labview instrumentation.

The experiment ran under small internal *AC* potential to generate the magnetic field in CMOS microcoil arrays, within a range of frequency from 1 Hz to 10 kHz. Afterwards, the results of the process were monitoring and plotting for each as well. The process starts by monitoring the control sensor, which is a bar of electrode immersed in the solution, then after the sensing layer that is immobilizing antibody on the surface of it. Then a combination of the biological cells and the magnetic bead got stable under magnetic field applied B > 0 as demonstrated in Figure 5-31. After removing the magnetic field; B = 0 also the results recorded as well, as demonstrated in Figure 5-32. Each status was plotting using Bode plot, magnitude of impedance vs. frequency, the result of this experiment shown in Figure 5-46.

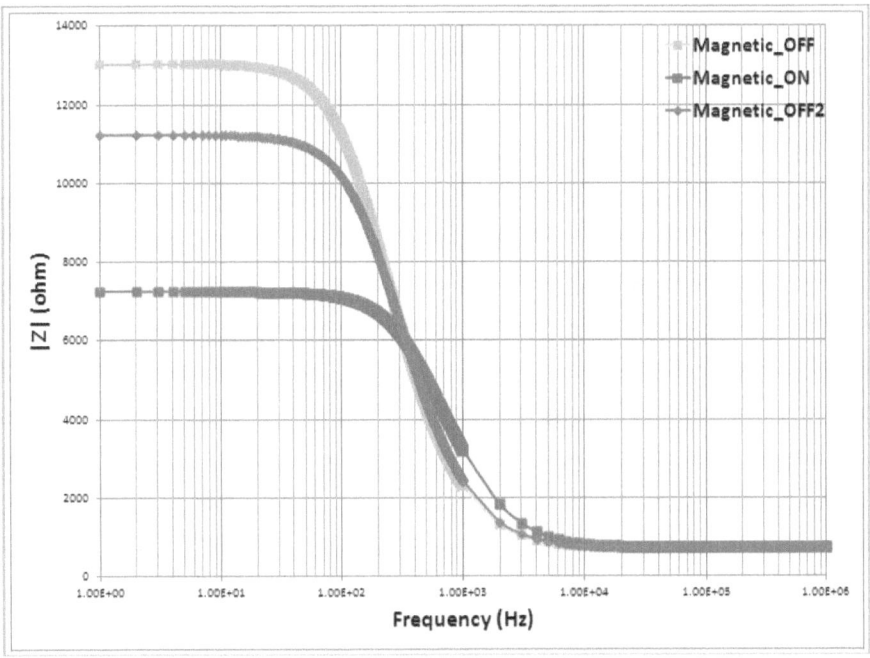

Figure 5-46 The experimental run for the entire process, control and sensing sensor before and after applying magnetic field.

In the case of the control sensor, the surface of IDMA not functionalized where the sensing layer, the IDMA functionalized as shown in Figure 5-30. Immobilization the antibody onto the surface of the working electrode (*WE*) should take place first follow then immersed *"WE"* into LB media that mixed with biological cells and magnetic bead to be attached.

As a result, the immunoreaction that took place in between immobilized antibodies and biological cells binding along with the magnetic bead were monitoring and recording for carrying out the difference in charge-transfer resistance R_{ct} and the double layer capacitance; C_{dl}, before and after applying the magnetic field. Figure 5-46 shows impedance measurements for both biosensors; control and functionalized. The control biosensor, which referred to it on the figure by the green line and signs, it has no modification to the surface of microelectrodes; called bare electrodes, therefore, the impedance shows the maximum due to the low concentration of the biological attached to the surface and the "Magnetic OFF". The functionalized biosensor where the antibodies immobilized on the surface of microelectrodes, there are two curves, the red line when the "Magnetic ON", and the blue line when the "Magnetic OFF2", the impedance shows the minimum for the case when the "Magnetic ON" and higher for the case when the magnetic released. However, the latter case still lesser than the control biosensor due the residual of the biological on the surface after releasing the magnetic field. As aforementioned in section 4.8.1 a layer that would reduce the moving and transferring charges in between the electrodes can create because of antibodies immobilization onto the electrode surface that means increasing the R_{ct} resistance. Consequently, this leads mainly to the basic rule that is saying the higher biological cells that bonded to the surface of the electrodes the higher double layer capacitance at low frequency range the minimum impedance measured.

The mechanism of the charge-transfer resistance (R_{ct}) and the double layer capacitance variations can confine due to the surface modifications during the immobilization of antibodies by always taking into account the frequency range. For the high concentration of binding biological cells associating with magnetic bead on the immobilized antibody electrode surface change the permittivity of the media in between the electrode fingers, which leads to change the double layer capacitance; accordingly. Where the surface modification of the microelectrodes under any circumstances such as the immobilization of antibodies and binding biological cells does not show significant variation on the Warburg impedance; Z_w and the solution resistance, R_{sol} as discussed in section 4.7.

5.7.4   Summary

CMOS microcoil-based system specifically designed, fabricated, and experimentally validated for realizing a new generation of multi-labs on a single chip (MLoC) System. CMOS-microcoil-based electrochemical impedance measurements incorporates hybrid microfluidic channel and IDMA combines the manipulation of paramagnetic microparticles (magnetic beads) through a magnetic field was employing for rapid detection of biological cells where with antibodies bound to the biosensor and magnetic bead surfaces. The integrated sensor is as a part of MLoC chip worked successfully and provided enhancements in the current magnetic system to impart robustness and improve the system performance when compared to other techniques. IDMA technology with a potential integrated within microfluidic channel (MFC) for biomedical and life sciences applications is the main valuable outcome within reach of miniaturization of biosensors that is improving the transducer sensitivity and selectivity.

As stated, the definition of originality aforementioned in "*section* 1.4", the CMOS microcoil techniques fill in the first and the third categories where the ideas have been previously published. The design in the literature made of a die within 2.0 *mm x* 3.0 mm using electroplating techniques but the tools for MLoC system are definitely different. In this design, the technology that used is CMOSP35; the area of the entire planar microcoil is 248.05 μm x 246.725 μm. The magnetic source is built using 32 microcoils in 4 x 8 arrays. Each coil, which made of three metals; M1, M2, and M3, connecting in series with vias. The integrated system described has an enormous potential to concentrate and enhance bacterial capture from samples. Moreover, this part of MLoC system fills also in the third category of originality, where the entire sensor implemented on-chip includes the IDMA sited on the top of the microcoils for magnetic field manipulation. The area of the IDMA sites in a 215.075 μm long and 114.775 μm width is placed. Each finger has 0.6 μm width and space, and 188.6 μm long. The IDMA design offers increased sensitivity to redox cycles, improving as the electrode gap decreases. Therefore, this integration should improve the detection limit by several orders of magnitude, shorten the analysis time and reduce non-specific detection events. The work includes two types of IDMA; on-chip using CMOS technology for CMOS Microcoil sensor and OFF-chip on MFCI surface using soft photolithograph technique inside the cleanroom. The digital circuits include the control circuit to steer the direction and the magnitude of the electrical current in the selected row of the microcoil array, which will reduce the fan-in of the entire chip. The lateral size of the MLoC chip is 2.23 by 3.04 mm^2 and the supply voltage is V_{dd} = 3.3 V.

5.8   References

[1]   Z. Hugh Fan, Shakuntala Mangru, Russ Granzow, Paul Heaney, Wen Ho, Qianping Dong, and Rajan Kumar, "Dynamic DNA Hybridization on a Chip Using Paramagnetic Beads", pp 4851-4859, September 28, 1999.

[2]   Mirowski, Elizabeth; Moreland, John; Russek, Stephen E.; Donahue, Michael, "Integrated microfluidic microfluidic isolation platform for magnetic particle manipulation in

biological systems", J. Applied Physics Letters, Vol. 84 Issue 10, p1786-1788, 3p, 2 diagrams; August 3, 2004.

[3]   Murat K. Yapici, Ali E. Ozmetin, Jun Zoua, Donald G. Naugle, "Development and experimental characterization of micromachined electromagnetic probes for biological manipulation and stimulation applications", Sensors and Actuators A 144, 213-221, 2008.

[4]   U. Lehmann, M. Sergio, S. Pietrocola, C. Niclass, E. Charbon, M.A.M. Gijs, "A CMOS Microsystem Combining Magnetic Actuation and in-Situ Optical Detection of Microparticles, Transducers 2007.

[5]   G. Friedman, B. Yellen, "Magnetic separation, manipulation and assembly of solid phase in fluids", Current Opinion in Colloid & Interface Science, Volume 10, Issues 3-4, Pages 158-166, October 2005.

[6]   Mark A. Hayes, Nolan A. Polson, Allison N. Phayre, and Antonio A. Garcia, "Flow-Based Microimmunoassay", Anal. Chem., 73, pp 5896-5902, November 10, 2001.

[7]   Stefan Miltenyi, Werner Müller, Walter Weichel, Andreas Radbruch, "High gradient magnetic cell sorting with MACS", Cytometry, 11, 231-239, 1990.

[8]   M.A.M. Gijs (MARTIN), "Magnetic Particle Handling in Lab-on-a-Chip Microsystems", in: Magnetic Nanostructures in Modern Technology, Bruno Azzerboni, Giovanni Asti, Luigi Pareti, Massimo Ghidini, page: 153-165, Microfluid Nanofluid, 1, 22-40, 2004.

[9]   K. Smistrup, B. G. Kjeldsen, J. L. Reimers, M. Dufva, J. Petersen and M. F. Hansen, "On-chip magnetic bead microarray using hydrodynamic focusing in a passive magnetic separator", Lab on a Chip, 5, 1315-1319, 2005.

[10]   K. Smistrup, T. Lund-Olesen, M.F. Hansen, P.T. Tang, "Microfluidic magnetic separator using an array of soft magnetic elements", J. Appl. Phys. 99, 08P102, 2006.

[11]   Furlani, É.p., "Magnetophoretic separation of blood Cells at the Microscale", Journal of Physics D: Applied Physics 2007: 40 (5) 1313-1319, 2007.

[12]   Jin-Woo Choi, Trifon M. Liakopoulos, Chong H. Ahn, "An on-chip magnetic bead separator using spiral electromagnets with semi-encapsulated permalloy", Biosensors and Bioelectronics, Volume 16, Issue 6, Pages 409-416, August 2001.

[13]   Ahn, C.H.; Allen, M.G.; Trimmer, W.; Jun, Y.-N.; Erramilli, S., "A fully integrated micromachined magnetic particle separator", Microelectromechanical Systems, Journal of Volume 5, Issue 3, Page(s):151-158, Sept. 1996.

[14]   Kristian Smistrup, Ole Hansen, Henrik Bruus, Mikkel F. Hansen, "Magnetic separation in microfluidic microfluidic systems using microfabricated electromagnets—experiments and simulations", Journal of Magnetism and Magnetic Materials, Volume 293, Issue 1, Pages 597-604, May 2005.

[15]   Liu, C., Lagae, L., Wirix-Speetjens, R., Borghs, G., "On-chip separation of magnetic particles with different magnetophoretic mobilities", Journal of Applied Physics, 101(2), art.nr. 024913,2007.

[16]   Zung-Hang Wei, Chiun-Peng Lee, Mei-Feng Lai, "Magnetic particle separation using controllable magnetic force switches", Journal of Magnetism and Magnetic Materials, Volume 322, Issue 1, Pages 19-24, January 2010.

[17]   X.-B. Wang, Y. Huang, F. F. Becker, and P. R. C. Gascoyne, "A unified theory of dielectrophoresis and travelling wave dielectrophoresis," J. Phys. D, Appl. Phys., vol. 27, pp. 1571-1574, 1994.

[18]   Hakho Lee, Yong Liu, Eben Alsberg, Donald E. Ingber, Robert M. Westervelt, Donhee Ham, "An IC/Microfluidic Hybrid Microsystem for 2D Magnetic Manipulation of

Individual Biological Cells", 2005 IEEE International Solid-State Circuits Conference, ISSCC 2005.

[19]   Lee, Hakho, "Microelectronic/microfluidic microfluidic hybrid system for the manipulation of biological cells", Ph.D. book, Harvard University, 150 pages; AAT 3194427, 2005.

[20]   Hakho Lee, Yong Liu, Robert M. Westervelt, and Donhee Ham, "IC/Microfluidic Hybrid System for Magnetic Manipulation of Biological Cells", IEEE Journal of Solid-State Circuits, Vol. 41, NO. 6, JUNE 2006.

[21]   Osamu Niwa, Yan Xu, H. Brian Halsall, William R. Heineman, "Small-volume voltammetric detection of 4-aminophenol with interdigitated array electrodes and its application to electrochemical enzyme immunoassay, pp 1559-1563, June 1993.

[22]   Osamu Niwa, Masao Morita, Hisao Tabei, "Electrochemical behavior of reversible redox species at interdigitated array electrodes with different geometries: consideration of redox cycling and collection efficiency", pp 447-452, March 1990.

[23]   Jennifer H. Thomas, Sang Kyung Kim, Peter J. Hesketh, H. Brian Halsall, and William R. Heineman, "Bead-Based Electrochemical Immunoassay for Bacteriophage MS2", pp 2700-2707, April 20, 2004.

[24]   Jin-Woo Choi, Kwang W. Oh, Jennifer H. Thomas, William R. Heineman, H. Brian Halsall, Joseph H. Nevin, Arthur J. Helmicki, H. Thurman Henderson, Chong H. Ahn, "An integrated microfluidic microfluidic biochemical detection system for protein analysis with magnetic bead-based sampling capabilities", Lab On a Chip, 2, 27 - 30, 2002.

[25]   C.S. Lee, H. Lee, R. M. Westervelt, "Microelectromagnets for the control of magnetic nanoparticles", Appl. Phys. Lett. 79 (20), 3308-3310, 2001.

[26]   Hakho Lee, Yong Liu, Donhee Ham, Robert M. Westervelt, "Integrated cell manipulation system-CMOS/microfluidic microfluidic hybrid", Lab On a Chip, 7, 331-337, 2007.

[27]   Lehmann, U.; Vandevyver, C.; Parashar, V.K.; DeCourten, D.; Gijs, M.A.M., "Two-dimensional magnetic droplet manipulation platform for miniaturized bioanalytical applications", Micro Electro Mechanical Systems, 2007. MEMS. IEEE 20th International Conference on 21-25 Jan. 2007 Page(s):521-524, 2007.

[28]   Heng-Ming Hsu, "Investigation on the layout parameters of on-chip inductor", Microelectronics Journal 37, 800-803, 2006.

[29]   D. Trumbull, I.K. Glasgow, D.J. Beebe, R.L. Magin, "Integrating microfabricated fluidic systems and NMR spectroscopy", IEEE Trans. Biomedical Eng., 47, 3-7, 2000.

[30]   L. Berry, L. Renaud, P. Kleimann, P. Morin, M. Armenean, H. Saint-Jalmes, "Development of implantable detection microcoils for minimally invasive NMR spectroscopy", Sensors and Actuators A: Physical, Volume 93, Issue 3, Pages 214-218, 15 October 2001.

[31]   L. Renaud, M. Armenean, L. Berry, P. Kleimann, P. Morin, M. Pitaval, J. O'Brien, M. Brunet, H. Saint-Jalmes, "Implantable planar RF microcoils for NMR microspectroscopy", Sensors and Actuators A: Physical, Volume 99, Issue 3, Pages 244-248, 5 June 2002.

[32]   Craninckx, J.; Steyaert, M.S.J.; "A 1.8-GHz low-phase-noise CMOS VCO using optimized hollow spiral inductors", Solid-State Circuits, IEEE Journal of Volume 32, Issue 5, Page(s):736-744, May 1997.

[33]   Sertac Eroglu, Barjor Gimi, Brian Roman, Gary Friedman, Richard L. Magin, "NMR Spiral Surface Microcoils: Design, Fabrication, and Imaging", Concepts in Magnetic Resonance Part B (Magnetic Resonance Engineering), Vol. 17B(1) 1-10, 2003.

[34]   B. Razavi, "Challenges in the Design of Frequency Synthesizers for Wireless Applications", Proc. CICC, pp.395-402, May 1997.

[35]   CMOS PLLs and VCOs for 4G Wireless, Ch5 pp. 17

[36]   J. Craninckx, Michiel Steyaert, "Wireless CMOS Frequency Synthesizer Design", the International Series in Engineering and Computer Science, Kluwer Academic, Netherland, 1998.

[37]   Lopez-Villegas, J.M.; Samitier, J.; Cane, C.; Losantos, P.; "Improvement of the quality factor of RF integrated inductors by layout optimization", Radio Frequency Integrated Circuits (RFIC) Symposium, 1998 IEEE, Page(s):169-172, 7-9 June 1998.

[38]   C. Massin, G. Boero, F. Vincent, J. Abenhaim, P. -A. Besse, R. S. Popovic, "High-Q factor RF planar microcoils for micro-scale NMR spectroscopy", Sensors and Actuators A: Physical, Volumes 97-98, Pages 280-288, 1 April 2002.

[39]   J. Long and M. Copeland, 'The modeling, characterization, and design of monolithic inductors for silicon RF IC's,"IEEE J. Solid-State Circuits, vol. 32, pp. 357-369, Mar. 1997.

[40]   J. N. Burghartz, D. C. Edelstein, K. A. Jenkins, and Y. H. Kwark,"Spiral inductors and transmission lines in silicon technology using copper damascene interconnects and low-loss substrates," IEEE Trans. Microwave Theory Tech., vol. 45, pp. 1961-1968, Oct. 1997.

[41]   A. C. Reyes, S. M. El-Ghazaly, S. J. Dorn, M. Dydyk, and D. K. Schroder, "Coplanar waveguides and microwave inductors on silicon substrates," IEEE Trans. Microwave Theory Tech., vol. 43, pp. 2016-2022, Sept. 1995.

[42]   J. Y.-C. Chang, A. A. Abidi, and M. Gaitan, "Large suspended inductors on silicon and their use in a CMOS RF amplifier," IEEE Electron Device Lett., vol. 14, pp. 246-248, May 1993.

[43]   C. P. Yue and S. S. Wong, "On-chip spiral inductors with patterned ground shields for Si-based RF IC's,"IEEE J. Solid-State Circuits, vol. 33, pp. 743-752, May 1998.

[44]   IC Layout Basics - A Practical Guide p138

[45]   J.M. Lopez-Villegas, J. Samitier, C. Cane, P. Losantos, J. Bausells, "Improvement of quality factor of RF integrated inductors by layout optimization", IEEE Trans. Microw. Theory Tech. 48, 76-83. 2000.

[46]   Lopez-Villegas, J.M.; Sieiro, J.; "Modeling of integrated inductors and transformers for RF applications", Thermal, Mechanical and Multi-Physics Simulation and Experiments in Micro-Electronics and Micro-Systems, 2005. EuroSimE 2005, Page(s):19-23, Proceedings of the 6th International Conference on 18-20 April 2005.

[47]   H.-M. Hsu, "Analytical formula for inductance of metal of various widths in spiral inductors", IEEE Trans. Electron Dev. 51, 1343-1346, 2004.

[48]   Yong Liu, Hakho Lee, Robert M. Westervelt, Donhee Ham, "CMOS -Based Magnetic Cell Manipulation System", in: CMOS.Biotechnology, ch.5, pp103, 2007.

[49]   Vermeiren, W., Straube, B.; Holubek, A., "Defect-oriented experiments in fault modelling and fault simulation of microsystem components", European Design and Test Conference, 1996. ED&TC 96. Proceedings, Page(s):522-527, 11-14 March 1996.

[50]   Chong H. Ahn; Allen, M.G., "Micromachined planar inductors on silicon wafers for MEMS applications", Industrial Electronics, IEEE Transactions on Volume 45, Issue 6, Page(s):866-876, Dec. 1998.

[51]   Greenhouse, H.; "Design of Planar Rectangular Microelectronic Inductors", Parts, Hybrids, and Packaging, IEEE Transactions on Volume 10, Issue 2, Page(s):101-109, Jun 1974.

[52]   Oshiro, O.; Tsujimoto, H.; Shirae, K.; A novel miniature planar inductor Magnetics", IEEE Transactions on Volume: 23, Issue: 5, Page(s): 3759 - 3761, 1987.

[53]   Ahn, C.H.; Allen, M.G., "A fully integrated micromachined magnetic particle manipulator and separator", Micro Electro Mechanical Systems, 1994, MEMS '94, Proceedings, IEEE Workshop on, Page(s):91 - 96, 25-28 Jan. 1994.

[54]   Baltes, H.P.; Popovic, R.S, "Integrated semiconductor magnetic field sensors", Proceedings of the IEEE, Volume 74, Issue 8, Page(s):1107-1132, Aug. 1986.

[55]   Manaresi, N.; Romani, A.; Medoro, G.; Altomare, L.; Leonardi, A.; Tartagni, M.; Guerrieri, R., "A CMOS Chip for Individual Cell Manipulation and Detection," IEEE J. Solid-State Circuits, vol. 38, no. 12, pp. 2297-2305, 2003.

[56]   Y. Huang, X.-B. Wang, J. A. Tame, R. Pethig, "Electrokinetic behavior of colloidal particles in travelling electric fields: Studies using yeast cells," J. Phys. D, Appl. Phys., vol. 26, pp. 1528-1535, 1993.

[57]   Brown, Robert, "A brief account of microscopical observations made in the months of June, July and August, 1827, on the particles contained in the pollen of plants; and on the general existence of active molecules in organic and inorganic bodies." Phil. Mag. 4, 161-173, 1828.

[58]   Einstein, A., "Investigations on the Theory of Brownian Movement". New York: Dover, 1956.

[59]   J. Dechow, A. Forchel, T. Lanz, A. Haase, "Fabrication of NMR microsensors for nanoliter sample volumes", Microelectronic Engineering, 53, Issues 1-4 517-519, June 2000.

[60]   Jin-Woo Choi, Chong H. Ahn, Shekhar Bhansali, H. Thurman Henderson, "A new magnetic bead-based, filterless bio-separator with planar electromagnet surfaces for integrated bio-detection systems", Sensors and Actuators B:

Chemical, Volume 68, Issues 1-3, Pages 34-39, 25 August 2000.

[61] Ahn, C.H.; Allen, M.G.; "Fluid micropumps based on rotary magnetic actuators", Micro Electro Mechanical Systems, MEMS '95, Proceedings. IEEE, Page(s):408, 2 Feb. 1995.

[62] Neamen, A. Donald, "Electronic Circuit Analysis and Design", 2nd, McGraw Hill, 2001.

[63] S. Eroglu, G. Friedman, R.L. Magin "Estimate of losses and signal-to-noise ratio in planar inductive micro-coil detectors used for NMR", IEEE Trans. Mag., Vol. 37, no. 4, part I, pp. 2787-2789, July 2001.

[64] Peck T. L.; Magin R. L.; Lauterbur P. C, "Design and analysis of microcoils for NMR microscopy", Journal of magnetic resonance, vol. 108, no2, pp. 114-124 Series 1995.

[65] Vesselle, H.; Collin, R.E.; "The signal-to-noise ratio of nuclear magnetic resonance surface coils and application to a lossy dielectric cylinder model. I. Theory", Biomedical Engineering, IEEE Transactions on Volume 42, Issue 5, Page(s):497-506, May 1995.

[66] Grant, Samuel; Friedman, Gary; Growney, Eric; Magin, Richard; "Signal-To-Noise Improvement with Multilayered Rf Microcoils", the 40th Experimental Nuclear Magnetic Resonance Conference, Orlando, FL. February 28 - March 5, 1999.

[67] Vesselle, H., Collin, R.E., "The signal-to-noise ratio of nuclear magnetic resonance surface coils and application to a lossy dielectric cylinder model. II. The case of cylindrical window coils", Biomedical Engineering, IEEE Transactions on Volume 42, Issue 5, Page(s):507 - 520, May 1995.

[68] Behrooz Fateh, "Modeling, Simulation and Optimization of a Microcoil for MRI-Cell Imaging", November 2006.

[69]   Hakho Lee, Donhee Ham, Robert M. Westervelt, "CMOS Biotechnology", Ch. 5, 6: design of the CMOS IC chip, page: 92, 116, Springer, 2007.

[70]   Paleček, E.; Fojta, M., "Magnetic beads as versatile tools for electrochemical DNA and protein biosensing", Talanta 2007: 74(3) 276-290, 2007.

[71]   Suk-Heung Song, Bong-Seop Kwak, Jae-Sung Park, Woochul Kim, Hyo-IL Jung, "Novel application of Joule heating to maintain biocompatible temperatures in a fully integrated electromagnetic cell sorting system", Sensors and Actuators A: Physical, Volume 151, Issue 1, Pages 64-70, 8 April 2009.

[72]   Ryan Marek, Michael Caruso, Abdolmohamad Rostami, Judith. B. Grinspan, Jayasri Das Sarma, "Magnetic cell sorting: A fast and effective method of concurrent isolation of high purity viable astrocytes and microglia from neonatal mouse brain tissue", Journal of Neuroscience Methods, Volume 175, Issue 1, 30 October 2008, Pages 108-118.

[73]   Zhijuan Cao, Zengxi Li, Yujie Zhao, Yumin Song, Jianzhong Lu, "Magnetic bead-based chemiluminescence detection of sequence-specific DNA by using catalytic nucleic acid labels", Analytica Chimica Acta, Volume 557, Issues 1-2, Pages 152-158, 31 January 2006.

[74]   Yonghao Zhang, Pinar Ozdemir, "Microfluidic DNA amplification-A review", Analytica Chimica Acta, Volume 638, Issue 2, Pages 115-125, 13 April 2009.

[75]   Andreas Thiel, Alexander Scheffold, Andreas Radbruch, "Immunomagnetic cell sorting-pushing the limits", Immunotechnology, Volume 4, Issue 2, Pages 89-96, October 1998.

[76]   Andreas Radbruch, Diether Recktenwald, "Detection and isolation of rare cells", Current Opinion in Immunology, Volume 7, Issue 2, Pages 270-273, April 1995.

[77]   Rolando Guidelli, Giovanni Aloisi, Lucia Becucci, Andrea Dolfi, Maria Rosa Moncelli, Francesco Tadini Buoninsegni, "Bioelectrochemistry at metal_water interfaces", Journal of Electroanalytical Chemistry, Volume 504, Issue 1, Pages 1-28, 4 May 2001.

[78]   Wan-Chi Lee, Kang-Yi Lien, Gwo-Bin Lee, Huan-Yao Lei, "An integrated microfluidic microfluidic system using magnetic beads for virus detection", Diagnostic Microbiology and Infectious Disease, Volume 60, Issue 1, Pages 51-58, January 2008.

[79]   Mamas I. Prodromidis, "Impedimetric immunosensors—A review", Electrochimica Acta, In Press, Corrected Proof, Available online 7, February 2009.

[80]   Eric Bakker and Martin Telting-Diaz, "Electrochemical Sensors", Anal. Chem., 2002, 74 (12), pp 2781-2800, May 07, 2002.

[81]   F. Patolsky, B. Filanovsky, E. Katz and I. Willner, "Photoswitchable Antigen-Antibody Interactions Studied by Impedance Spectroscopy", J. Phys. Chem. B, 102, 10359-10367 (1998).

[82]   Ivo Šafařík, Mirka Šafaříková, "Use of magnetic techniques for the isolation of cells", Journal of Chromatography B: Biomedical Sciences and Applications, Volume 722, Issues 1-2, Pages 33-53, 5 February 1999.

[83]   W.S. Prestvik, A. Berge, P.C. Mork, P.M. Stenstad, J. Ugelstad, "Preparation And Application of Monosized Magnetic Particles In Selective Cell Separation", in: U. Hafeli, W. Schutt, J. Teller, M. Zborowski (Eds.), Scientific and Clinical Applications of Magnetic Carriers, Plenum Press, New York, London, 11-35, 1997.

[84]   F.-L. Zhan, L.-M. Kuo, W.-Y. Chang, S.-W. Wang, Chih-Heng Lin, Y.-S. Yang, and Michael S.-C. Lu, "An Electrochemical Dopamine Sensor with CMOS Detection

Circuit," 6th IEEE Int. Conf. on Sensors, Atlanta, USA, pp. 1448-1451, Oct. 28-31, 2007.

[85]   Stephen Nussey, Saffron, "Whitehead Ligand binding to hormone receptors", in Endocrinology: An Integrated Approach, Published by BIOS Scientific Publishers Ltd. ISBN 1-85996-252-1, Vol. 9 2001.

[86]   X.J.A. Janssen, L.J. van IJzendoorn, M.W.J. Prins, "On-chip manipulation and detection of magnetic particles for functional biosensors", Biosensors and Bioelectronics, Volume 23, Issue 6, Pages 833-838, 18 January 2008.

[87]   Liju Yang, Yanbin Li, Carl L. Griffis, Michael G. Johnson, "Interdigitated microelectrode (IME) impedance sensor for the detection of viable Salmonella typhimurium", Biosensors and Bioelectronics, Volume 19, Issue 10, Pages 1139-1147, 15 May 2004.

[88]   Madalina Tudorache, Michelle Co, Henric Lifgren, and Jenny Emnéus, "Ultrasensitive Magnetic Particle-Based Immunosupported Liquid Membrane Assay", pp 7156-7162, October 14, 2005.

[89]   Qasem Ramadan, Victor Samper, Daniel P. Poenar, Chen Yu, "An integrated microfluidic platform for magnetic microbeads separation and confinement", Biosensors and Bioelectronics, Volume 21, Issue 9, Pages 1693-1702, 15 March 2006.

[90]   Ying Sun, Yuping Bai, Daqian Song, Xiaozhou Li, Liying Wang, Hanqi Zhang, "Design and performances of immunoassay based on SPR biosensor with magnetic microbeads", Biosensors and Bioelectronics, Volume 23, Issue 4, Pages 473-478, 30 November 2007.

[91]   Nicole Jaffrezic-Renault, Claude Martelet, Yann Chevolot, Jean-Pierre Cloarec, "Biosensors and Bio-Bar Code Assays Based on Biofunctionalized Magnetic Microbeads", Sensors 2007, 7(4), 589-614, 2007.

[92]   Daniel L. Graham, Hugo A. Ferreira, Paulo P. Freitas, "Magnetoresistive-based biosensors and biochips", Trends in Biotechnology, Volume 22, Issue 9, Pages 455-462, September 2004.

[93]   Kwang W. Oh, Chong H. Ahn, "Magnetic Actuation", Comprehensive Microsystems, Chapter 2.02, Pages 39-68, 2008.

[94]   Elizabeth Mirowski, John Moreland, Arthur Zhang, Stephen E. Russek, "Manipulation and sorting of magnetic particles by a magnetic force microscope on a microfluidic magnetic trap platform", Applied Physics Letters, 86, 243901, Jun 2005.

[95]   Gijs, M.A.M., "Magnetic particle handling microsystems for miniaturized analytical applications", Engineering in Medicine and Biology Society, 2007. EMBS 2007. 29th Annual International Conference of the IEEE, 22-26, Page(s):4088-4089, Aug. 2007.

[96]   J. Ugelstad, P. Stenstad, L. Kilaas, W. S. Prestvik, R. Herje, A. Berge, E. Hornes, "Monodisperse magnetic polymer particles. New biochemical and biomedical applications", Blood Purif, vol. 11, pp. 349-369, 1993.

[97]   G. T. Rado, H. Suhl, "Magnetism", vol. 3, New York: Academic Press, 1963.

[98]   U. Häfeli, "Scientific and clinical applications of magnetic carriers", New York: Plenum Press, 1997.

[99]   Jeffrey Travis, JimKring, "LabVIEW for Everyone: Graphical Programming Made Easy and Fun", Third Edition, July 27, 2006.

[100]   Krichevsky, A.; Smith, M. J.; Whitman, L. J.; Johnson, M. B.; Clinton, T. W.; Perry, L. L.; Applegate, B. M.; OConnor, K.; Csonka, L. N.; "Trapping motile magnetotactic bacteria with a magnetic recording head", Journal of Applied Physics Volume: 101, Issue: 1 2007, Page(s): 014701 - 014701-6.

[101] Xue-Mei   Li,   Xiao-Yan   Yang,   Shu-Sheng   Zhang,
       "Electrochemical enzyme immunoassay using model labels",
       TrAC Trends in Analytical Chemistry, Volume 27, Issue 6,
       June 2008, Pages 543-553.

[102] R. Afshar, Y. Moser, T. Lehnert, M.A.M. Gijs, "Magnetic
       particle dosing and size separation in a microfluidic channel",
       Sensors and Actuators B: Chemical, In Press, Corrected
       Proof, Available online 29 August 2009.

Chapter 6 - MLoC Insight

The researchers and biomedicine engineers would appreciate the final success of the MLoC system when they realize the capability of this system. The capability of the **MLoC** system complies with employing the advantages of miniaturization that converts the devices from macro scale to micro/nano scale resulting in reduced diffusion lengths and minimized geometries. The miniaturization reduces the cost and time, which helps increase the manufacturing that pushes forward the research and the development in the area of life science and biomedicine applications.

In terms of the transduction techniques used, the four main classes of biosensors that lead to a new generation of multi-labs-on-a-single chip (MLoC) contains capacitive, optical, Electrochemical Impedance Spectroscopy (EIS) and planar microcoils for magnetic field generation techniques.

The first of the four techniques, the CMOS CBCM capacitive system had a drawback that was the limited detection level of the pathogens (around 12 pF). To overcome this problem, a single processing unit was added to the CBCM technique. The signal-processing circuit aims to convert the current passing through the output stage into a digital signal, where the frequency is proportional to the concentration of the pathogens in medium. This is solved by using a hybrid analog/digital integration scheme. In this circuit, an analog integrator and a discriminator convert the current generated as byproduct into a train of digital pulses; current-to-frequency converter (CFC). The CBCM technique passed the validation procedures successfully and its profile that was obtained matched the hypobook.

As for the optical biosensor, its surface was increased to the VPNP phototransistor 32 x 32 arrays instead of 16 x 16 arrays, in the light of the fact that the sensitivity of the optical sensor depends on the exposed area to the light. In addition, the chip contains all the required resistors on-chip. The device passed the validation procedures and it passed the experimental procedures that were performed from low to high concentration of bacteria on this device specifically.

The electrochemical impedance spectroscopy (EIS) has all of its stages implemented on-chip including the voltage controller and signal-processing unit along with their associating capacitors and resistors. The system passed the validation tests and a profile resulted as expected from the sensor as a part of the MLoC system.

As for the CMOS Microcoil biosensors technique, the entire sensor implemented on-chip includes the IDMA sited on top of the microcoils for magnetic field manipulation. This system ran perfectly and the manipulation on the sensing surface where the magnetic particle was located was performed by observing the variation of the impedance of the output. The aforementioned approaches (the CBCM, Optical and EIS methods) required sample pre-treatment steps and signal amplification strategies, which caused some complications and challenges. The CMOS microcoil solved both challenges at once through the manipulation of the magnetic particles on the sensing layer in addition to the contamination problem that the CBCM and the microfluidic channel were suffering from. This technique will leave the sensors clean and reusable.

The two types of IDMA; the on-chip using CMOS technology for planar CMOS Microcoil sensor and the OFF-chip on MFCI surface using soft photolithography technique inside the cleanroom were helpful and significantly aided the MLoC system to come to the light and bring the results as expected.

The experimental set-up has a key role in running the MLoC system. The Labview code that was written especially for this system was as a definite bonus in making the experimental set-up easier and let the MLoC system come to the light as a new generation.

All the aforementioned biosensors worked separately as expected and successfully passed all the validation tests. However, the chip is able to run more than one experiment using the different techniques if a multiplexer is added to the interface of the MLoC system. This could be considered as a future work suggestion.

The recent MLoC system is still suffering from off-chip components that should be added to make the system fully IC. In the future, all of these external components can be added on-chip and implemented on-chip as well. The MLoC system can be updated to a more efficient system through adding a wireless unit on board and receiving the data off the chip by a special receiver. An EDP technique is one of the more common techniques that are widely used but it is not available on the MLoC and it can be added to the MLoC system for it to become more comprehensive and integrated.

Appendix-A   List of Tables

Appendix-B   List of Figures

Appendix-C List of symbols

APS: Active-Pixel-Sensor
BEC: Bioelectrochemistry
BOD: Biological Oxygen Demand
CBCM: Charge Based Capacitance Measurement
CCDs: Charge-Coupled Devices
CE: Capturing Efficiency
CE: Counter Electrode
CFU: Colony Forming Units
CL: Chemiluminescence
CMOS: Complementary Metal Oxide silicon
CNT: Carbon Nanotube
COC: Cyclic Olefin Copolymer
CPE: Constant Phase Element
CVC: Current-Voltage Converter
DAMP: Differential amplifier
DAQ: Data acquisition devices
ECL: Electrochemiluminescence
EIS: Electrochemical Impedance Spectroscopy
ELISA: Enzyme-Linked Immunosorbent Assay
ELONA: Enzyme Linked Oligonucleotide Assay
EM: Electromagnetic
FISH: Fluorescence In Situ Hybridization
GFP: Green Fluorescent Protein
GL: Gouy layer
GPIB: General Purpose Interface Bus
HER2:   Human Epidermal growth factor Receptor 2

HL: Helmholtz double layer
IBH: Infectious Brain Homogenate
IDMA: Interdigitated Microelectrodes Array
Ig: Immunoglobulin: Ig
IMEA: Immunomagnetic Electrochemical Assay
ISFET: Ion-Sensitive Field-Effect Transistor
Labview: Laboratory Virtual Instrument Engineering Workbench
LB: Luria-Bertani
LCE: Low Capture Efficiency
LIF: Laser-Induced Fluorescence
LoC: Laboratory-on-Chip
LOD: Limit of Detection
MDS: Minimum Detectable Signal
MEMS: MicroElectroMechanical Systems
MFC: Microfluidic channel
μTAS: Micro Total Analysis Systems
MIM: Metal-Insulator-Metal
MLoC: Multi-Lab-On-A-Chip
MMCC: Metal-Metal Comb-Capacitors
MR: Magnetic Resonance
MRM: Magnetic Resonance Microscopy
MRM: Magnetic Resonance Microscopy
NADH: Nicotinamide Adenine Dinucleotide
NMR: Nuclear Magnetic Resonance
OCP: Open Circuit Potential
OFS: Optical Fluorescence Spectroscopy
OS: Optical spectroscopy
PBP: Pre-Bake Process
PDEIS: Potentiodynamic Electrochemical Impedance
            Spectroscopy
PDMS: PolyDiMethylSiloxane
PIN: Positive-Intrinsic-Negative (PIN) photodiode

PLOC: Polymer Lab-On-A-Chip
PMFC: Polymer Microfluidic Chip
PMMA: Polymethyl-Methacrylate
PMP: Paramagnetic Particles
PMT: Photomultiplier Tube
POCT: Point-Of-Care Testing
PT: Phototransistor
RE: Reference Electrode
RF: Radio Frequency
RGA: Regulated Gain Amplifier
SCCA: Squamous Cell Carcinoma Antigen
SCR: Space-Charge Region
SEJ: Silicon and Electrolyte Junction
SNR: Signal-To-Noise Ratio
SPR: Plasmon Resonance
SQUID: Superconducting Quantum Interference Device
SS: Surface States
TIA: Trans-Impedance Amplifier
VCOs: Voltage-Controlled Oscillator
VI: Virtual Instruments
VISA: Virtual Instrument Software Architecture
VLSI: Very Large Scale Integrated
VPNP: Vertical P-N-P transistor
VPTA: Vertical Phototransistor Array
WE: Work Electrode
WEC: Working Electrode Collector
WEG: Working Electrode Generator
ZIF: Zero Insertion Force

Appendix-D Labview Programming and Source Code

D1. Labview Programming

Front page

Page 1

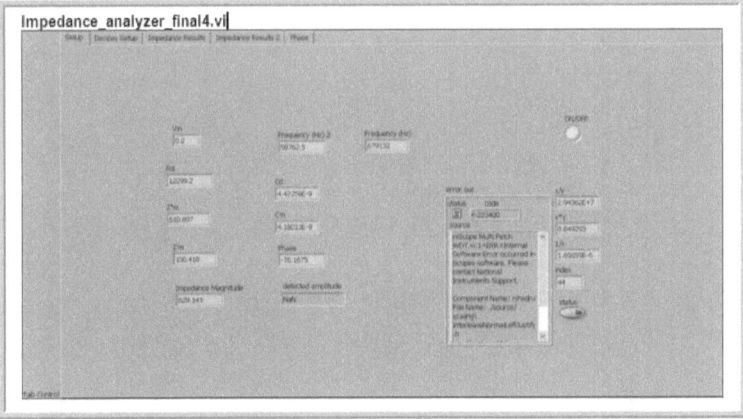

Page 2

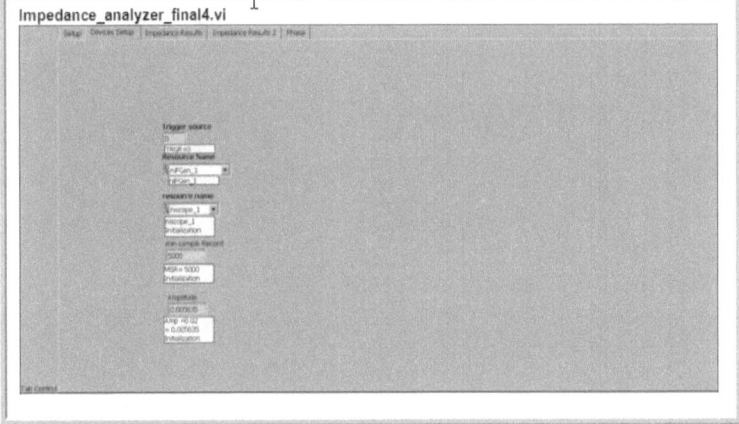

Page 3

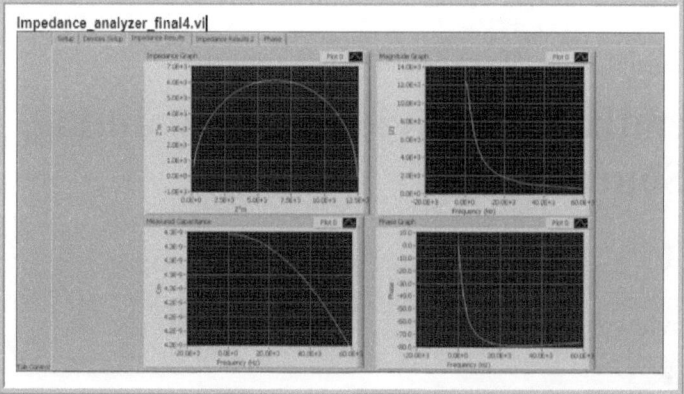

Page 4

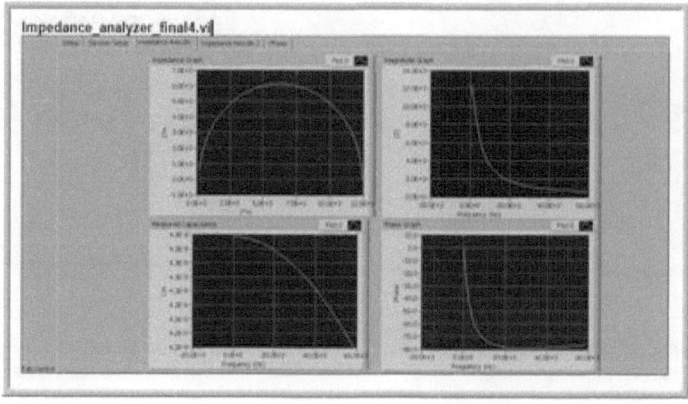

Page 5

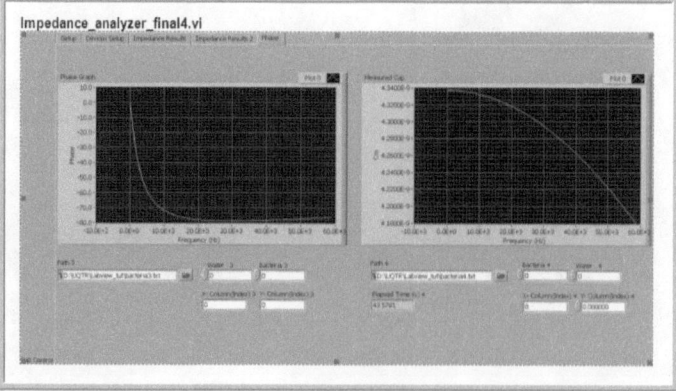

D2. Icons and Descriptions

 Elapsed Time4

Elapsed Time: Indicates the amount of time that has elapsed since the specified start time.

This Express VI is configured as follows: Time Target: 0.001 s Auto Reset: Off

 Convert to Dynamic Data2

Convert to Dynamic Data: Converts numeric, Boolean, waveform and array data types to the dynamic data type for use with Express VIs.

 Write To Measurement File

Write To Measurement File: Writes data to a text-based measurement file (.lvm) or binary measurement file (.tdm). This Express VI is configured as follows: Mode: Save to one file. Filename: D:\UQTR\Labview_tut\Cm.tdms If a file already exists: Append to file

 Merge Errors.vi

C:\Program Files\National Instruments\LabVIEW 8.2\vi.lib\Utility\error.llb\Merge Errors.vi

 niScope Configure Trigger Edge.vi

C:\Program Files\National Instruments\LabVIEW 8.2\instr.lib\niScope\Configure\Trigger\ niScope Configure Trigger Edge.vi

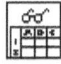 Read From Spreadsheet File (DBL).vi

C:\Program Files\National Instruments\LabVIEW 8.2\vi.lib\Utility\file.llb\Read From Spreadsheet File (DBL).vi

 Read From Spreadsheet File.vi

C:\Program Files\National Instruments\LabVIEW 8.2\vi.lib\Utility\file.llb\Read From Spreadsheet File.vi

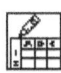 Write To Spreadsheet File (string).vi

C:\Program Files\National Instruments\LabVIEW 8.2\vi.lib\Utility\file.llb\Write To Spreadsheet File (string).vi

 Write To Spreadsheet File (DBL).vi

C:\Program Files\National Instruments\LabVIEW 8.2\vi.lib\Utility\file.llb\Write To Spreadsheet File (DBL).vi

Write To Spreadsheet File.vi

C:\Program Files\National Instruments\LabVIEW 8.2\vi.lib\Utility\file.llb\Write To Spreadsheet File.vi

 niScope Close.vi

C:\Program Files\National Instruments\LabVIEW 8.2\instr.lib\NISCOPE\niScope Close.vi

 niFgen Close.vi

C:\Program Files\National Instruments\LabVIEW 8.2\instr.lib\niFgen\niFgen.LLB\niFgen Close.vi

 NI_MAPro.lvlib:Extract Single Tone Information 1 Chan.vi

C:\Program Files\National Instruments\LabVIEW 8.2\vi.lib\measure\matone.llb\Extract Single Tone Information 1 Chan.vi

 NI_MAPro.lvlib:Extract Single Tone Information.vi

C:\Program Files\National Instruments\LabVIEW 8.2\vi.lib\measure\matone.llb\Extract Single Tone Information.vi

 WDT Index Channel DBL.vi

C:\Program Files\National Instruments\LabVIEW 8.2\vi.lib\Waveform\WDTOps.llb\WDT Index Channel DBL.vi

 Index Waveform Array.vi

C:\Program Files\National Instruments\LabVIEW 8.2\vi.lib\Waveform\WDTOps.llb\Index Waveform Array.vi

 niScope Abort.vi

C:\Program Files\National Instruments\LabVIEW 8.2\instr.lib\niScope\Acquire\Fetch\niScope Abort.vi

 niScope Multi Fetch WDT.vi

D:\UQTR\Labview_tut\niScope Multi Fetch WDT.vi

niScope Fetch (poly).vi

C:\Program Files\National Instruments\LabVIEW
8.2\instr.lib\niScope\Acquire\Fetch\niScope Fetch (poly).vi

 niScope Initiate Acquisition.vi

D:\UQTR\Labview_tut\niScope Initiate Acquisition.vi

 niFgen Initialize.vi

D:\UQTR\Labview_tut\niFgen Initialize.vi

 niScope Commit.vi

C:\Program Files\National Instruments\LabVIEW
8.2\instr.lib\niScope\Utility\niScope Commit.vi

 niScope Configure Trigger (poly).vi

C:\Program Files\National
Instruments\LabVIEW8.2\instr.lib\niScope\Configure\Trigger\niScope Configure
Trigger (poly).vi

 niScope Configure Horizontal Timing.vi

C:\Program Files\National
Instruments\LabVIEW8.2\instr.lib\NISCOPE\Configure\Horizontal\ niScope
Configure Horizontal Timing.vi

 niScope Configure Chan Characteristics.vi

C:\Program Files\National Instruments\LabVIEW
8.2\instr.lib\NISCOPE\Configure\Vertical\ niScope Configure Chan
Characteristics.vi

 niScope Configure Vertical.vi

C:\Program Files\National Instruments\LabVIEW
8.2\instr.lib\NISCOPE\Configure\Vertical\ niScope Configure Vertical.vi

 niScope Initialize.vi

D:\UQTR\Labview_tut\niScope Initialize.vi

niFgen Configure Output Mode.vi

C:\Program Files\National Instruments\LabVIEW
8.2\instr.lib\niFgen\niFgen.LLB\niFgen Configure Output Mode.vi

 niFgen Configure Standard Waveform.vi

C:\Program Files\National Instruments\LabVIEW
8.2\instr.lib\niFgen\niFgen.LLB\niFgen Configure Standard Waveform.vi

 niFgen Initiate Generation.vi

C:\Program Files\National Instruments\LabVIEW
8.2\instr.lib\niFgen\niFgen.LLB\niFgen Initiate Generation.vi

 niFgen Commit.vi

C:\Program Files\National Instruments\LabVIEW
8.2\instr.lib\niFgen\niFgen.LLB\niFgen Commit.vi.

D3: Block diagram

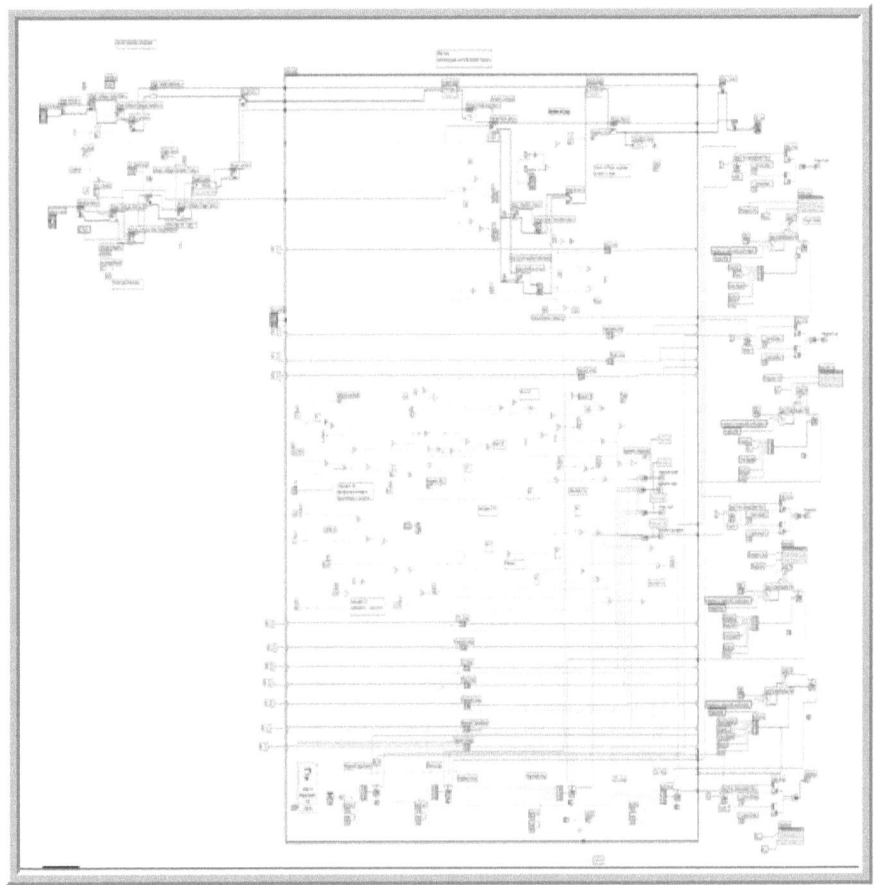

Index